Control of Human Reproduction

MONOGRAPHS FOR STUDENTS OF MEDICINE

SERIES EDITORS

Professor R. J. Harrison, F.R.S., M.D., D.Sc.,
School of Anatomy, University of Cambridge, Cambridge

Professor A. W. Asscher, M.D., F.R.C.P.
K.R.U.F. Institute of Renal Disease, Welsh National School of Medicine, Cardiff

MONOGRAPHS FOR STUDENTS OF MEDICINE

CONTROL OF HUMAN REPRODUCTION

R. L. HOLMES, M.Sc., M.B., Ch.B., Ph.D., D.Sc.

and

C. A. FOX, M.A., M.D., L.R.C.P., M.R.C.S., M.R.C.G.P., F.P.A.Cert.

Department of Anatomy, University of Leeds

1979

ACADEMIC PRESS

London   New York   San Francisco

A Subsidiary of Harcourt Brace Jovanovich, Publishers

ACADEMIC PRESS (LONDON) LTD.
24-28 Oval Road,
London, NW1

United States Edition published by
ACADEMIC PRESS INC.
111 Fifth Avenue
New York, New York 10003

Library of Congress Catalog Card Number: 78-75273
ISBN: 0-12-353450-X

PRINTED IN GREAT BRITAIN BY THE LAVENHAM PRESS LIMITED
LAVENHAM, SUFFOLK

Preface

The endocrinology of reproduction has many features common to all vertebrates. Most notable of these is probably the dominant part played by the pituitary gland acting as an intermediary between the central nervous and reproductive systems. Between species however, even closely related ones, there are often considerable variations in such aspects as the patterns of reproductive activity, the influences exerted by environmental factors and the relative importance of the various organs involved. Relatively few species have been subjected to extensive study; among mammals these are mainly the common laboratory animals and those of commercial importance. Extrapolation from observations on one species to others less intensely studied, even if closely related, is fallible and it is particularly unwise to assume that findings in animals can be applied directly to man, in whom "experimental" studies are necessarily largely confined to observations of normal, therapeutic and pathological aspects of reproductive processes.

A general pattern of the role played by the endocrine system in reproductive processes has emerged from the vast number of studies which have been reported; but the complexity and variability within the field of study means that inevitably generalisations introduce errors. Hence, this attempt to present a general survey, with particular reference to Man, includes statements which are not universally applicable, and which are either incorrect as regards some species, or do not accord with the views of one or other authority. It is hoped that the short list of references and suggestions for further reading, by and large restricted to reviews, may direct the reader to the greater precision (and complexity) of original studies.

The thanks of the authors are due to Professor R. J. Harrison, F.R.S. for his careful reading of the text and valuable comments; to Mr. Anthony Watkinson of Academic Press for his patience and help; and to Mrs. Barbara Whitehead for her secretarial skills.

R.L.H.
C.A.F.

Contents

1

Introduction

The various secretory tissues of the body which are commonly considered to make up the endocrine "system" have in common the essential characteristic that they secrete into the blood physiologically active substances, hormones, which exert an influence on the activity of other tissues, often situated in some other parts of the body. Endocrine glands have a rich blood supply and lack a system of ducts; but both structurally and functionally they are diverse. In general the effect of their secretions is relatively long-lasting by comparison with, for example, the action of neuro-transmitter substances, whose short-term activity is usually localized to the synaptic regions of neurons or the neuro-muscular junctions formed by motor end plates.

In so far as reproduction involves not only the reproductive organs but virtually the whole individual, the entire endocrine system is concerned in the process, but some of its components are more directly involved than others. Leading roles are played by the hypothalamus and the pituitary gland and by the gonads, the testes in the male and the ovaries in the female. The hypothalamus and pituitary together form a complex hormone-secreting control mechanism which is essential, not only for reproduction, but for the activity of other endocrine glands and for many aspects of metabolism. The gonads have dual roles, acting as endocrine glands secreting male (androgens) and female (oestrogens and progesterone) sex hormones, as well as producing the male and female germ cells, spermatozoa and ova, respectively.

The adrenal (suprarenal) glands are also of considerable importance in reproductive activity. The adrenal cortex secretes a number of steroid hormones concerned in metabolism and among these are adrenal androgens and oestrogens. Other endocrine glands influence the reproductive system to a lesser extent. The hormones of the thyroid gland are particularly involved in general metabolism, but under or over-secretion can have important effects on developmental and reproductive processes. In recent years the pineal body (or gland), whose function was uncertain for a long time, has been shown to be capable of influencing some aspects of reproductive cycles.

HORMONES

The hormones most directly concerned with reproductive processes act in several ways. In both men and women the pituitary gland secretes two gonadotropins, which act on the testes or ovaries and control not only the development of the spermatozoa and ova, but also the growth and secretion of

1

endocrine cells lying within these organs. These produce steroids, which in turn act on the reproductive tracts, controlling their growth and the exocrine secretions of intrinsic and accessory glands, such as the endometrial glands in the lining of the uterus and the seminal vesicles which in the male contribute to the seminal fluid. The gonadal steroid hormones take part in complex feedback mechanisms which modulate the secretion of the pituitary gonadotropins (see p. 18).

Anterior Pituitary Hormones

The pituitary gland secretes at least nine distinct hormones; seven of these come from the anterior pituitary (the adenohypophysis) and two from the posterior (neurohypophysis). Six of the adenohypophysial ones are secreted by the part of the gland called the pars distalis, whose structure is described on p. 12, and three of these are of particular importance in reproduction, namely:

follicle stimulating hormone (FSH), which brings about maturation of the ovarian follicles and, in the male, influences spermatogenesis;

luteinizing hormone (LH) which with FSH effects ovulation, and subsequently growth and secretion of the corpus luteum; in the male this hormone stimulates the activity of the testicular interstitial tissue which secretes androgens (see p. 97); hence it is sometimes referred to as "interstitial cell stimulating hormone" (ICSH), but to avoid confusion the term LH is used throughout the text;

lactotropic hormone (LTH) or prolactin, which plays a part in the development and maintenance of the secretion of milk by the mammary glands.

The three other hormones of the pars distalis are particularly involved in general metabolic processes, the first two acting via the target endocrine glands. They are:

adrenocorticotropic hormone (ACTH), which controls the growth and secretory activity of the cortex of the adrenal (suprarenal) glands;

thyrotropic hormone (TSH), which controls growth and secretory activity of the thyroid gland;

somatotropic (or growth) hormone (STH) whose action is not confined to any specific target organs but has a widespread influence on metabolic processes and growth.

All these hormones are protein or peptide in nature. The gonadotropic hormones FSH and LH, and TSH are glycoproteins, that is their molecules have a carbohydrate and a protein component. This characteristic is shared by a hormone produced by the placenta, human chorionic gonadotropin (HCG) (see p. 57). Each of these four hormones is made up of two sub-units, called alpha and beta, the alpha units being homologous for all four hormones, the beta ones hormone-specific. If the original molecule of hormone is broken down to the two sub-units, each of these is found to have generally a low biological activity, but high activity is restored if the two are reunited.

The seventh hormone of the anterior pituitary is secreted by cells of the pars intermedia (see p. 13), a part of the gland which is present in most mammals, but ill-developed or, according to some, absent in man. The hormone, intermedin, can however be extracted from human pituitaries. It occurs in at least two chemical forms, and a part of the molecule is structurally common to this hormone and to ACTH, with which it shares some actions. Although many effects of intermedin have been described in man and in animals its role is unclear. In many species, particularly fish, amphibia and reptiles, intermedin acts directly on pigment cells: hence its alternative name of melanocyte or melanophore-stimulating hormone and the common abbreviation of this to MSH.

Posterior pituitary hormones

The posterior or neural part of the pituitary gland (see p. 11) of man and mammals secretes two hormones, antidiuretic hormone (ADH), which is sometimes called vasopressin, and oxytocin. These are both designated as neurosecretory hormones, since they are elaborated by neurons situated in the hypothalamus. From here they pass along nerve fibres to the posterior part of the pituitary gland where they are stored, bound to carrier substances called neurophysins. Each of these hormones is an octapeptide, containing two linked molecules of the sulphur-containing amino acid cysteine, the two usually considered as constituting one molecule of cystine. The arrangement of the amino acids in the molecule of oxytocin is shown in Fig. 1. The

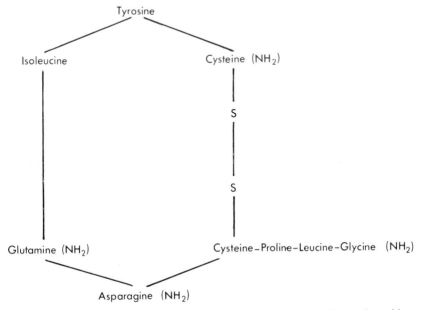

Fig. 1. Structure of a molecule of oxytocin to show the arrangement of the amino acids.

structure of ADH differs in that arginine replaces leucine in the side chain, and phenylalanine replaces isoleucine in the ring.

Oxytocin increases the contractility of smooth muscle of the reproductive tract. It is reflexly secreted during coitus and causes contractions of the uterine muscle which may aid the passage of spermatozoa through the reproductive tract and increase the likelihood of fertilisation. During labour (parturition) oxytocin stimulates uterine contractions and aids delivery of the fetus: and in the period of lactation following the birth of the infant the hormone is reflexly released during suckling and, by bringing about contraction of myoepithelial cells and smooth muscle in the mammary glands assists the outflow of milk.

ADH is not directly concerned in reproductive processes. Its main action is to increase the absorption of water from the distal renal tubules and collecting ducts, so that a concentrated urine is secreted from the kidneys. It owes its alternative name, vasopressin, to its ability to increase the blood pressure, but this effect is usually of secondary importance. The close chemical similarity of ADH and oxytocin is reflected in the finding that each can to a small extent exert the effects of the other.

Gonadal hormones

The "sex" hormones are commonly thought of as being either "male", secreted by the testes or "female", by the ovaries. The testicular hormones, androgens, include the primary hormone testosterone, while those coming from the ovaries include oestrogens and progesterone. Both male and female gonads however can synthesise both "male" and "female" hormones and, although in normal individuals the hormones of the appropriate sex predominate, both types occur in the blood of men and women and as breakdown products in their urine. Futhermore, both "male" and "female" hormones are synthesised in the adrenal cortex of each sex.

The gonadal hormones share a common basic chemical structure with others which are largely produced by the adrenal cortex and also by the liver. These are all classified as steroids. Those which are secreted by the testis and ovary influence particularly the reproductive system, as indeed do androgenic and oestrogenic steroids arising in the adrenal glands. Many of the adrenal steroids however are primarily involved in general metabolic processes in tissues not primarily concerned with reproductive activity. Some steroids of adrenal and of gonadal origin, notably androgens, exert a protein anabolic effect; that is they bring about retention of nitrogen and an increased synthesis of protein. This effect is not confined to the reproductive system, but occurs in tissues of the body such as bones, kidney and notably skeletal muscle. The increased muscular development following the administration of anabolic steroids has been made use of to increase the muscularity and performance of athletes and to increase the meat yield of cattle.

The basic structure of steroids is a nucleus of 17 carbon atoms, conventionally numbered as in Fig. 2, the valence bonds for each carbon being to adjacent carbon atoms or to hydrogen. The presence of methyl (CH3) groups or more elaborate side chains in different compounds, and the addition of oxygen to form —OH or =O at variously positioned carbon atoms of the basic nucleus, may profoundly modify the activity of a steroid. Such additional carbon atoms are also numbered, so that compounds with 18, 19 or more basic carbon atoms occur (Fig. 2).

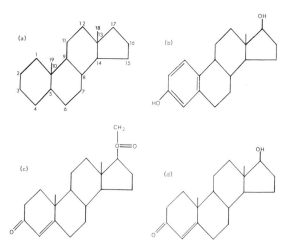

Fig. 2. Diagram to show (a) the conventional numbering of the carbon atoms in the steroid nucleus; (b) structure of oestradiol; (c) progesterone; (d) testosterone.

The precise role of any given steroid is often difficult to assess, for many of them have both specific effects exerted on particular organs and tissues and more general influences on some aspects of metabolism. Furthermore the response of a given tissue to a hormone varies and is influenced by genetic, nutritional, endocrine and other factors. Many different steroids can be isolated from tissues; and while some of these are intermediaries in the synthesis of a given end product such as testosterone, they themselves commonly have inherent endocrine activity. The lack of clear cut distinction between "male" and "female" steroid hormones is further emphasised by the fact that oestrogens and progesterone occur as intermediate products in the synthesis of androgens, and androgens are produced in the synthesis of oestrogens.

Biosynthesis and metabolism of steroids

Large amounts of steroids are synthesised by the adrenal cortex, testis and ovary, all of which have the enzymes necessary for the elaboration of the hormones from two-carbon acetate. Normally any one of these tissues produces a predominance of steroids with a particular range of actions, although each is capable of producing virtually any type. Thus the adrenal cortex usually secretes a variety of corticoids involved in general metabolic process, and some androgens; the testis secretes mainly androgens and the ovary mainly oestrogens and progesterone. But in abnormal states the secondary products may become the predominant ones.

The basic step in the synthesis of steroids by living tissues is the transformation of two-carbon acetate ($CH_3COO—$) into cholesterol. Not all tissues are able to utilise this two-carbon compound, and some require more complex blood-borne precursors. This applies to the placenta, which can use only small amounts of acetate for the synthesis of progesterone, and to the liver. Such tissues are in this sense incomplete endocrine organs, depending on substances formed by adrenal cortex, testis and ovary for the synthesis of their own highly active steroids; but given these "pre-hormones", which often have a relatively low activity, both liver and placenta can produce potent substances.

It is then hardly surprising that large numbers of steroids can be isolated from steroid-producing tissues and from blood. Some of these are potent substances known to be essential factors in metabolic and reproductive functions while others, formed as intermediaries in the synthetic processes, do not necessarily have such essential roles. For example, a basic pathway for the synthesis of oestrogens involves the formation of progesterone and androgens, as in the scheme.

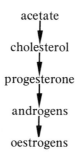

The most active naturally occurring oestrogen, oestradiol, can be formed by the sequence

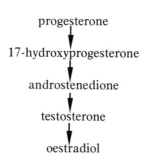

a process which involves the formation as intermediaries of the weak androgen, androstenedione, and the potent one, testosterone. An alternative sequence, giving oestrone as the end product, begins with pregnenolone

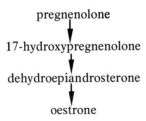

The metabolism of steroids takes place in the liver but also in many other tissues. Structural changes such as reduction of double bonds and oxidation results in diminution of their activity, and conjugation with sulphate or glucuronate occurs. Conjugated metabolites are excreted in the urine; metabolites of progesterone include pregnanediol and 17-hydroxyprogesterone; oestrogens are excreted as conjugated substances, and androgens as 17-ketosteroids.

Mode of Action of Sex Hormones

Testosterone, the most potent circulating androgen, is transported in the blood free or loosely bound to carrier proteins. These are beta-globulins know as sex hormone binding globulin (SHBG) and testosterone binding globulin (TeBG). Levels of these globulins are raised during pregnancy and by ingestion of oestrogens (including most oral contraceptives); increases are also seen in hyperthyroidism, hepatic cirrhosis and male hypogonadism. Androgens and oestrogens compete for binding sites on these globulins, and any increase favours the binding of androgens. This results in a fall in the level of free-circulating testosterone and a rise in the available oestrogen. Such a situation is thought to explain the gynaecomastia exhibited in the conditions mentioned.

In considering the action of steroid hormones at the cellular level it is important to understand the current nomenclature. A *target cell* is one proved by bioassay procedures to be under the regulation of a given type of steroid hormone. A *receptor* is an intracellular protein component responsible for the specific and high-affinity binding of a particular hormone and playing an integral part in its mechanism of action. An *acceptor is* a nuclear component responsible for the high affinity but limited retention of a steroid hormone-receptor complex in chromatin.

The entry of testosterone through the target cell membrane is facilitated by the action of cyclic-AMP (adenosine-3,5-cyclic monophosphate). Within the target cell it is metabolised by the enzyme 5-alpha reductase to the powerful androgen 5-alpha dihydrotestosterone which is thought to be the active androgen at the cellular level. The dihydrotestosterone-receptor protein complex is available for reaction with nuclear acceptor sites in the chromatin. At the nuclear level DNA acts as a template for the androgenic response through the accepted ribosomal RNA and messenger RNA mechanisms. The whole process is reversible so that the receptor protein-androgen complex does not form covalent bonds with the nuclear acceptor components. The antiandrogen action of oestrogens and cyproterone acetate may be considered in terms of competition for receptor binding sites at the target cell.

As already noted, the anabolic action of testosterone stimulates cell growth, increases body weight and causes nitrogen retention; additionally there is greater secretion of sebum and accelerated bone maturation. Thus, administration of anabolic steroids to children of small stature can be counter-productive by causing earlier fusion of epiphyses.

Measurement of hormones in the blood

The original bioassay methods depended on the growth of the comb in caponised cocks or increase in size of the rat ventral prostate. Analytical methods were gradually perfected so that sample size of 50 ml plasma, for example, using paper chromatography followed by enzymic conversion of the recovered testosterone to oestradiol which was measured fluorimetrically, was eventually reduced to 2 ml for competitive protein binding assays. The introduction of the radioimmunoassay has allowed the analysis of several hundred samples of less than 1 ml in a few days.

Radioimmunoassay depends on the competition between radioactively labelled hormone and unlabelled hormone for specific sites of an antibody specific to the hormone under investigation. The antibody is produced in an animal to which the antigen is foreign. The higher the blood concentration of unlabelled hormone, the less radioactive labelled hormone will be bound to antibody. It is possible to separate bound from free hormone and to measure the quantity of labelled hormone associated with bound antibody. A standard curve is prepared using known quantities of hormone and the concentration of hormone in an unknown sample may be read directly off the curve. It is assumed that antibody-bound hormone is completely separated from free hormone and that the radioactivity is measured in antibody-bound hormone. The normal values for plasma testosterone are 3-11 ng/ml in the male and 0.2-0.5 ng/ml in the female.

Oestrogens may be measured by chemical methods such as fluorimetry or gas chromatography but the preliminary purification which is so necessary for these techniques has proved tedious and time consuming. Here again, radioimmunoassay has great advantages and some centres are claiming reliable results. Plasma levels of 17-beta oestradiol vary around a mean of 50 ng/ml at mid-cycle reaching a nadir at the menstrual flow.

For the investigator, the change from large sample size taking perhaps a week for a few results to the modern situation of small volume multiple sample analysis has opened new vistas.

Pheromones

These can be considered to come under the broad heading of "hormones". They are chemical substances which typically bring about integration of activities among individuals of the same species, and their effects are particularly marked in invertebrates. Originally called ectohormones, they differ from the substances commonly classed as hormones in that the recipients respond to substances liberated by other individuals rather than to their own internal secretions. Minute amounts of pheromones are detectable by chemoreceptors. Their actions are particularly evident in invertebrates, in which they can for example initiate or inhibit complex developmental processes, or induce behaviour associated with reproductive activity. Female silkworm moths and cockroaches release substances which, as sex attractants, direct males to the females often over long distances and also trigger male sexual behaviour.

A well known example of a pheromone is "queen-bee substance". This, of known chemical structure, is secreted by mandibular glands of the queen; when ingested by the workers it inhibits development of their ovaries. Pheromones also act in some vertebrates and influence reproductive processes in some mammals (see p. 129).

2

The Pituitary Gland and Hypothalamus

Development and parts

This gland, which is often called the hypophysis, lies in the sella turcica, a bony fossa in the base of the skull (Fig. 3). This fossa has a roof of dura mater, called the diaphragma sellae, through which passes the pituitary stalk which connects the gland to the overlying hypothalamus. The stalk is attached to a swelling on the basal aspect of this part of the brain, the tuber cinereum.

The pituitary is made up of two main parts, the adenohypophysis and the neurohypophysis. These are derived embryologically from different sources. The adenohypophysis is formed from Rathke's pouch, a diverticulum from the roof of the future pharynx which extends up towards the overlying neural tube. The neurohypophysis develops from a hollow downgrowth of this tube which is closely applied to the posterior wall of Rathke's pouch (Fig. 4). Thus, the adenohypophysis, which in man forms the anterior part of the gland, is of epithelial origin and when fully developed remains an epithelial secretory organ. The neurohypophysis forms the posterior part of the gland, and remains an essentially neural structure.

Rathke's pouch and the neural downgrowth are present in human embryos of about 3mm. At first the lumen of the pouch is continuous with the cavity of the pharynx, but soon this continuity is lost by obliteration of the lower (juxta-pharyngeal) part of the lumen, leaving an upper hollow epithelial part which is for a time joined by a strand of epithelial cells to the epithelium of the pharynx. Later this strand disappears, but commonly a few cells persist just deep to the pharyngeal epithelium and form a "pharyngeal hypophysis", later separated from the main gland by development of the bony base of skull. The infundibular downgrowth also has a lumen, continuous with the cavity of the neural tube: in many but not all species this disappears except for its upper part, and the human neurohypophysis is a solid structure.

The fully formed adenohypophysis consists of three parts, commonly designated as pars distalis, pars tuberalis and pars intermedia (Fig. 5). The pars distalis, which is sometimes called the pars anterior, is the largest of these, and develops as a thickening of the anterior wall of the epithelial Rathke's pouch. It secretes the six tropic hormones, FSH, LH, LTH, ACTH, TSH, and STH.

The pars tuberalis develops from two lateral buds which grow out from the

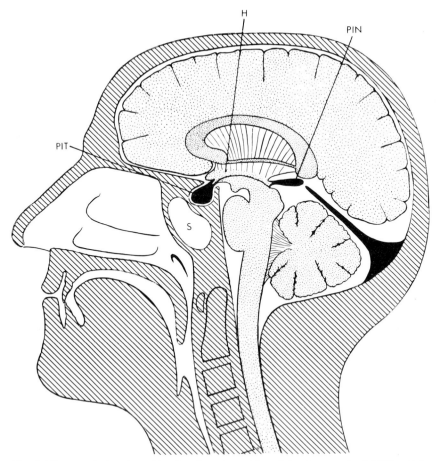

Fig. 3. Diagram of a hemisected head to show the position of the pituitary gland (PIT) and the pineal body (PIN). Central nervous tissue is shown in light stipple. (H-hypothalamus; S-sphenoidal air sinus).

upper anterior mass of adenohypophysial cells and fuse in the mid-line, closely applied to the stalk of the infundibulum and the tuber cinereum. In many species this forms a collar of cells around the stalk; the function of this part of the gland is not yet understood. The pars intermedia, which is well developed in lower mammals but not in man, arises from the posterior wall of the pouch closely applied to the neural downgrowth.

The neurohypophysis eventually differentiates into three parts (Fig. 5): the median eminence, which is a specialised vascular zone of the tuber cinereum of the base hypothalamus; the infundibular stem, a stalk of nerve fibres; and the infundibular process, which lies in the sella turcica and forms the "posterior" pituitary. The latter is the largest part of the neurohypophysis.

The three parts of the adenohypophysis are made up essentially of epithelial cells closely associated with blood vessels. In the pars distalis, the secretory cells are arranged in follicular groups separated by a small amount of connective tissue carrying the rich capillary bed which extends throughout this part of the gland.Classically the cells have been described as chromophils, which can be stained with a variety of dyes and chromophobes, which usually have a smaller amount of cytoplasm and stain poorly. Further differentiation can be made between the chromophils, since some of these have an affinity for basic dyes and are hence classed as basophils, while others take up acidic ones, such as eosin, and can be described as acidophils or eosinophils.

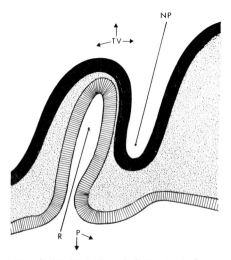

Fig. 4. Sagittal section through the developing pituitary gland of an early embryo. Rathke's pouch (R) at this stage has a lumen which communicates with the pharynx (P). The developing neurohypophysis (NP) also has a cavity continuous with that of the future third ventricle (TV). Note the close apposition of the epithelial (Rathke's pouch) and nervous components of the developing gland.

   Since this classification of the secretory cells was established by the latter half of the last century great progress has been made in the techniques available for the identification of types of cell.The use of more complex mixtures of dyes and histochemical methods made it possible to differentiate at least six types of secretory cell in the pars distalis. Electron microscopy has increased the accuracy of the identification of these types by various criteria, notably the size of their cytoplasmic granules. Techiques of ultracentrifugation have been used to obtain fractions of granules (and other cellular components) which can be studied by electron microscopy and also assayed for hormone activity, and the more recent technique of immunocytochemistry allows the identification of hormones in individual secretory cells.

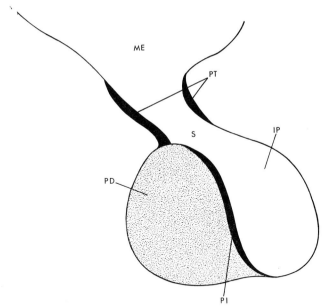

Fig. 5. Diagram of a mid-sagittal section through the pituitary gland to show its component parts. PD-pars distalis; PI-pars intermedia; PT-pars tuberalis; ME-median eminence of the tuber cinereum; S-pituitary stem (stalk); IP-infundibular process.

Thus, for some species at any rate, each tropic hormone can be associated with a distinct type of cell. Cells which secrete LTH and STH are both acidophilic, but their granules differ considerably in size (ca. 600 and 350 nm respectively). The two types of cell secreting FSH and LH both stain positively with the periodic acid-Schiff stain for mucoproteins, and both contain smaller granules; while TSH secreting cells, also PAS-positive, contain few small granules. Electron microscopy has also shown that chromophobes, which stain weakly and contain few granules, may be cells in an inactive state but that others , usually with abundant cytoplasm, may be in a state of hyperactivity. The latter stain poorly because they lack granules which, although still being produced, are not being stored but are leaving the cells as soon as they are formed. Cell of this type are found in certain kinds of pituitary tumours and may be associated with excess production of the relevant hormone.

The pars intermedia in most mammalian species commonly consists of several layers of cells closely applied to the infundibular process and usually separated from the pars distalis by the intraglandular cleft which represents a remnant of the lumen of Rathke's pouch. This part of the gland is relatively poorly vascularised. In man the pars intermedia persists only as a thin lamina of cells and colloid-filled cysts, and there is no intraglandular cleft; some authors indeed deny the existence of a pars intermedia in man. The pars tuberalis is made up of groups of cells among which lie numerous vessels connected with the portal vascular system (see below). The cells are largely chromophobic, but electron microscopy has shown that (in the rabbit) many contain small cytoplasmic granules. On the basis of immunohistochemical and extraction studies it has been suggested that some of the cells of the pars tuberalis contain LH.

By contrast with the adenohypophysis, the neurohypophysis is made up largely of the processes of hypothalamic nerve cells which, having traversed the median eminence and infundibular stem, end in enlargements closely associated with blood vessels in the infundibular process. Cells called pituicytes lie among the fibres. The infundibular process is not in itself a secretory structure in the sense of being responsible for the synthesis, storage and release of hormones, but acts chiefly as an organ of storage and release. Synthesis of its hormones occurs in the cell bodies of two paired groups of hypothalamic neurons, the supraoptic and paraventricular nuclei, and it is the processes of these cells which make up the bulk of the infundibular stem and process and transport the secretory material to the place of storage and release.

The neurohypophysis is an example of a "neurosecretory" system. Neurosecretion can be briefly described as the elaboration of hormonal substances by neurons and their release into the bloodstream from nerve terminals, with the additional criterion that the hormonal material, or some associated "carrier" substance, can be stained specifically for optical microscopy and can be detected by the electron microscope. Many authors distinguish between "neurosecretion" and the formation of "neurotransmitters" such as acetylcholine, which act only briefly and usually at their point of release.

Blood supply

The blood supply of the pituitary gland is of overwhelming importance not only for the normal metabolism of the gland, but also for its control by the nervous system. The supply to the adenohypophysis involves a "portal" system, in which blood does not pass directly from arteries to veins via a single capillary bed, but flows through two separate capillary networks which are linked by portal veins. The capillary bed which is directly supplied by arterioles is called the primary one, and that supplied by portal veins, the secondary.

In the hypothalamo-pituitary complex, the primary capillary network lies in the nervous tissue of the median eminence and, in some species, among the nerve fibres of the infundibular stem. Blood which has passed through these capillaries is collected into a number of portal veins or venules which run down the stem and open into the secondary capillary network in the pars distalis (Fig. 6) which it traverses before draining into the venous blood of the intracranial venous sinuses, thus regaining the systemic circulation. On a point of terminology, the infundibular *stem*, as used by some authors, refers only to the nerve fibres passing from the hypothalamus to the posterior pituitary, while *stalk* includes both these and the accompanying portal vessels.

The primary plexus in the median eminence and stalk is not a simple set of capillaries but a complex of short and long loops and, in larger mammals, vascular "spikes" (Fig. 6) which penetrate some distance (up to several millimetres in man) into the neural tissue. This region is a zone of neurovascular association in which nerve fibres from various regions of the hypothalamus end on these special capillary formations, which constitute the origin of the portal system. Specific chemical agents, called releasing factors or releasing hormones, are secreted by these nerve fibres into the blood circulating through the capillaries, and these substances are responsible for the control by the nervous system of secretory activity of the pars distalis. Release-inhibiting substances are also secreted (see p. 18). The neuro-secretory fibres passing from the supraoptic and paraventricular nuclei to the infundibular process traverse the median eminence

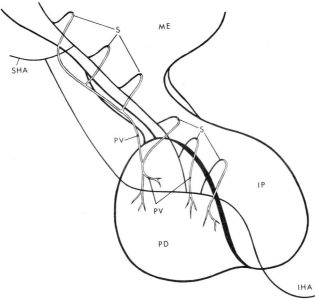

Fig. 6. Diagram to show the blood supply of the anterior pituitary. (SHA and IHA - superior and inferior hypophysial arteries; S-vascular spikes; PV-portal veins; ME-median eminence; PD-pars distalis; IP-infundibular process).

In mammals, including man, the arterial blood supply to the pituitary is derived from two sets of vessels, the superior and inferior hypophysial arteries, which themselves originate from the internal carotid arteries inside the cranial cavity. The infundibular process is largely supplied directly from the inferior hypophysial arteries, while the adenohypophysis (in particular the pars distalis) gets most of its blood from the superior vessels via the portal veins. In man some portal veins lying within the gland derive blood from primary capillary formations fed from the inferior hypophysial arteries (Fig. 6), so that the blood reaching the pars distalis comes from both superior and inferior hypophysial vessels. The portal veins carrying blood from the inferior arteries, which has passed through primary capillaries lying in the intra-glandular part of the stalk, are described as short portal veins, to distinguish them from the long portal veins which drain the primary plexus lying in the upper part of the neurohypophysis. The short portal veins supply blood to the more posterior (juxtaneural) part of the pars distalis, while the rest is supplied largely by the long vessels. This arrangement is of considerable importance in situations where there is a partial blockage or destruction of the portal veins: thus if only the veins arising in the upper part of the stalk are involved that part of the gland supplied by short portal vessels would still receive a blood supply and survive.

In many species, probably including man, the pars distalis receives no direct arterial blood supply and depends on the blood which reaches it via the portal vessels for all its requirements. Thus portal blood serves the function of supplying the gland with its metabolic needs and removing its waste products as well as carrying the chemical factors by means of which the central nervous system exerts control over the activity of this complex endocrine organ.

THE CONTROL OF PITUITARY ACTIVITY

A great many experimental studies, mainly carried out since the 1930s, have clearly shown that there is a special relationship between the pituitary gland and the hypothalamus, and that the anatomical situation of the gland and, particularly, its vascular connections with the median eminence, are essential for the normal functioning of the adenohypophysis. The development of current ideas was of necessity based to a large extent on experimental work carried out on animals. This enormous body of work enabled the formulation of principles which are largely applicable to the mechanisms of control of human reproductive activity. It was shown, for example, that the passage of an electric current through the head of an oestrous rabbit was followed by ovulation, indicating the release of gonadotropin. Electrical stimulation of the tuber cinereum or anterior hypothalamus also resulted in gonadotropin secretion, but direct stimulation of the pituitary gland itself did not. The central nervous system thus seemed to be involved in the secretory process.

Many experiments involved direct interference with the pituitary stalk. Transection of this divides both the nerve fibres and the portal vessels, and it was not easy to distinguish what effects might be due to damage to one or other of these structures. A further complication was the fact already noted that the portal vessels constitute the chief and in many species virtually the only blood supply to the pars distalis. Hence their interruption deprives this part of the gland of blood and leads to death of secretory cells and consequent deficiency of their endocrine secretions. We now know that there will also be the effects of loss of the hypothalamic releasing factors. Many conflicting reports of the results of such transection experiments were due to failure to appreciate that the portal vessels readily regenerate, so that unless some kind of barrier is placed between the cut ends of a transected stalk, an appreciable degree of revascularization of the gland can occur within a short time, and loss of anterior pituitary function may then be minimal. Hence the effect of transection of the pituitary stalk varied considerably.

The loss of the nutritional components of the portal blood can be offset to an appreciable extent by experiments in which the gland is removed from its position in the sella turcica and placed in some other site adjacent to vessels from which it can obtain a supply of "non-portal" blood adequate for the nourishment of the adenohypophysial cells. Experiments of this kind showed that even when the transplanted gland did acquire a good blood supply it failed to secrete the tropic hormones in anything but small amounts, with the exception of LTH. If such transplanted tissue was later replaced under the median eminence and acquired a blood supply from that source, secretory activity often returned; rats which had become anoestrous and sterile resumed oestrous cycles, and in some instances mated and became pregnant.

Releasing factors and releasing hormones

The pituitary gland thus seemed to differ from an endocrine gland such as the thyroid, which can continue to secrete if transplanted to a part of the body remote from its usual position. For many years it had been thought that the control of adenohypophysial activity was exerted by a direct innervation of the gland, and an apparent nerve supply to the secretory tissue had been described. Such observations proved to be largely in error and fine connective tissue fibres, which are readily revealed by many of the techniques used to show nerves, had been wrongly identified. Electron microscopy can more certainly differentiate between reticular and nerve fibres, and it now seems certain that there is no appreciable nerve supply to the pars distalis, although nerve fibres are present in the pars intermedia and pars tuberalis. As far as the pars distalis is concerned the essential link with the central nervous system is a vascular one, namely the pituitary portal system of vessels. As already noted, the blood passing to the pituitary via these vessels carries specific factors released into the capillaries of the primary plexus from hypothalamic nerve fibres, which control the release of tropic hormones from the cells of the adenohypophysis.

The correctness of the "releasing factor" hypothesis was indicated when it was shown that extracts of hypothalamic (median eminence) tissue could release FSH and LH from the pituitary. Similar studies for other tropic hormones suggested that the secretion of each was regulated by a specific factor. These were named according to their action and given appropriate abbreviations: FSH-releasing factor, FRF; LH-releasing factor, LRF; thyrotropin-releasing factor, TRF; corticotropin-releasing factor, CRF; and STH-releasing factor, commonly designated GRF.

The mechanism controlling the secretion of LTH (prolactin) appeared to differ from that for the other five hormones. It has already been noted that although a pituitary transplanted away from the median eminence secretes very small amounts of most of the tropic hormones, the secretion of LTH increases. This is because the hypothalamic factor normally controlling the secretion of this hormone has an inhibitory rather than a releasing effect, so that if pituitary tissue is removed from the portal blood supply which contains an appreciable amount of this inhibitory factor (named prolactin inhibitory factor, PIF), the secretion of LTH increases. An inhibitory factor for growth hormone has also been reported, so that GRF is partnered by an antagonistic GIF.

The secretion of MSH (intermedin) by the pars intermedia seems to be controlled in a similar way and both releasing and inhibiting factors (MRF and MIF) have been isolated. The presence of a nerve supply to this part of the gland allows the possibility of direct nervous control of its activity, so that unlike the pars distalis, a dual control mechanism, humoral and nervous, might be exerted over the pars intermedia.

Since the formulation of the hypothesis that chemical factors such as those described above were involved in hypothalamic control of adenohypophysial activity, hypothalamic extracts have yielded highly purified preparations, chemical analysis has been achieved and, in some instances, the substances have been synthesised. Once the chemical structure of any of these factors is known it is referred to as a hormone; hence the use of the terms "tropic hormone" releasing hormone, TH-RH. A further point of considerable importance is that strong evidence has been produced in favour of there being only one hypothalamic factor/hormone responsible for the secretion of the two pituitary hormones FSH and LH (see p. 35). This single hormone, which has been synthesised, is designated LH/FSH-RH. Recently it has been proposed that since these hypothalamic hormones control not only the release of tropic hormones but also their synthesis, they should be termed Regulating rather than Releasing hormones; but the same abbreviations can still be used.

Feedback mechanisms

There is now no doubt that the central nervous system directly controls secretory activity of the adenohypophysis via the portal vascular link. Even before the role of these blood vessels had been appreciated however it was realised that the secretory activity of some of the target organs controlled by the pituitary was "self regulating", and that the level of a hormone circulating in the blood could modulate the secretory activity of the cells producing it. This mechanism operates via the pituitary and involves changes in the output of tropic hormones. For example, the secretion of thyroxine by the thyroid gland is directly controlled by circulating TSH originating in the pars distalis; an increased output of TSH stimulates the thyroid gland to secrete more thyroxine, and a decrease has the opposite effect. Under normal conditions, however, the output of TSH from the pituitary is regulated by the amount of thyroxine in the blood: a high level acts to diminish the output of TSH, so that output of thyroxine from the thyroid gland decreases, while a low or falling level of thyroxine allows the secretion of TSH to increase and the trend is reversed (Fig. 7). This constitutes a negative feedback mechanism, in contrast to a positive one, in which an increase in secretion of a target gland hormone would result in an increase in the appropriate tropic hormone.

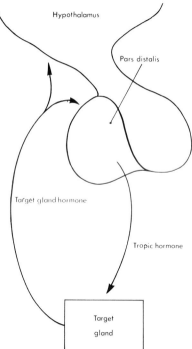

Fig. 7. Diagram to illustrate a simple negative feedback mechanism. The anterior pituitary tropic hormone stimulates a target gland to produce a hormone which acts on the hypothalamus/anterior pituitary to suppress the output of the tropic hormone.

Similar feedback mechanisms govern the secretory activity of other target organs—notably the testes, ovaries and adrenal cortex. In each of these systems, a tropic pituitary hormone acts on a specific target organ, whose secretory products in turn modulate the output of a tropic hormone. Such a clearly defined functional relationship does not apply when a tropic hormone, such as STH, acts more generally on metabolic processes rather than on a specific secretory organ.

Initially it was thought that feedback mechanisms involved a direct effect of target gland hormones on the anterior pituitary. When the dominant role played by the hypothalamus in pituitary activity was recognised, it was realised that the hypothalamus was likely to be involved in feedback effects. This has proved to be so, although some control may be exercised directly on the secretory cells of the gland and, in the case of the thyroid, this seems to be the most important mechanism.

Since the formulation of the role of simple negative feedback effects in the regulation of endocrine activity, it has become apparent that a much more complex mechanism obtains. "Long" feedback mechanisms such as those described coexist with "short" ones, in which the various tropic hormones themselves act on the hypothalamus. Two other mechanisms also have been described; one involves monitoring by the hypothalamus of the releasing factors which are being secreted into the portal blood; the other a direct regulation of the release of tropic hormones by their own concentration in tissues.

A further complication is that the effect of feedback is not necessarily constant. The steroid hormones secreted by the gonads may act in both negative and positive feedback mechanisms, and the hypothalamo-pituitary complex may vary greatly in its sensitivity to them at different times of life, and in different phases of reproductive activity. These aspects are discussed later in relation to puberty and menstrual cycles.

Finally it should be noted that feedback effects are not the only ones exerted by hormones on the central nervous system. The neural activity of areas both within and beyond the hypothalamus is influenced by androgens, oestrogens and other hormones which can modify developmental processes as well as functional and behavioural aspects of reproductive activity.

NEUROHYPOPHYSIAL HORMONES

An understanding of the relationship between the neurohypophysis and the hypothalamus was achieved earlier than for the adenohypophysis and largely stemmed from experimental studies in the 1930s, using monkeys. It was found that transection of the pituitary stalk gave rise to a severe disturbance of water metabolism, in which the animals excreted large amounts of very dilute urine. This condition, which is know as diabetes insipidus, occurs in man associated with damage to the hypothalamus and posterior pituitary. When the nerve fibres of the stalk are divided, that part of the neuro-hypophysis below the lesion degenerates, and changes also occur in the supraoptic and paraventricular neurons in the hypothalamus. Later studies showed that if radioactive cysteine (labelled with S^{35}) is injected into the cerebrospinal fluid of the ventricles it is quickly incorporated into these neurons, and subsequently the labelled material travels down the nerve fibres of the stalk, finally being stored in the infundibular process. The labelled amino acid is incorporated into the hormones ADH and oxytocin, which are elaborated in the neural cell bodies in the hypothalamus and bound to carrier substances (neurophysins).

The posterior pituitary is therefore concerned with the transport, storage and release of these hormones, not with their synthesis.

Release of neurohypophysial hormones

Release of ADH from the nerve fibres of the infundibular process occurs in response to a rise in the osmotic pressure of the plasma circulating through the hypothalamus. The hormone released into the bloodstream acts on the distal tubules and collecting ducts of the kidneys, increasing the amount of water reabsorbed from the urine, increasing its concentration and conserving water. A fall in the plasma osmotic pressure, such as follows the ingestion of water, results in a diminished secretion of ADH, and the excretion of a more dilute urine.

The release of oxytocin is brought about by a neural reflex, as for example when the child is put to the breast of a lactating woman. In this instance there is a rapid release of hormone from the posterior pituitary, which passes in the blood to the mammary tissue and there effects the contraction of myoepithelial and smooth muscle cells. Milk is thus actively expelled from the ducts of the breast and may even spurt from the nipple: this is known as the "let-down" of milk. Oxytocin is also released during labour, when it acts on the smooth muscle of the uterus.

3

Female Reproductive Cycles

Oestrous and menstrual cycles

Reproductive processes in living creatures conform to some kind of pattern, familiar, even to those who have no particular knowledge of biology, in the seasonal breeding habits of wild and domesticated creatures, the periodic onset of "heat" in pet female dogs and cats and in the menstrual cycles of women.

In the female of most species the successive periods of reproductive activity and quiescence are know as "oestrous" cycles; in each of these the animal passes from a state of reproductive quiescence, anoestrus, to one of activity, oestrus, which after successful mating will be followed by pregnancy. Oestrus is preceded by pro-oestrus, a phase of development of the reproductive organs to the oestrous state, and followed by met-oestrus, a phase of regression. Unsuccessful mating (and certain other kinds of stimuli) during oestrus may lead to a state of pseudopregnancy before the basic cycle is resumed.

In some species oestrous cycles only occur during a breeding season of limited duration, but in others they may, unless interrupted by pregnancy, extend throughout the year. Furthermore, the pattern of oestrous cycles varies greatly in different species of mammals. Some have a series of successive cycles and are classed as polyoestrous, while others have only one cycle in any one part of the year, and are classed as monoestrous. The time-scale of cycles varies greatly (Table I). In rats, for example, cycles may succeed one another at intervals as short as four or five days. In such polyoestrous animals the successive periods of oestrus are not separated by the return of the reproductive tract to the anoestrous condition, but rather by a short interphase, dioestrus.

Oestrous cycles have the following characteristics:
1. the female is usually sexually receptive only at the time of oestrus;
2. there is usually no bleeding from the uterus at any time during the cycle;
3. oestrus may be associated with external changes, such as the swelling of the perivaginal tissues;
4. ovulation, if spontaneous, occurs at the time of oestrus, and hence during the period of sexual receptivity.

In some species, for example, the ferret and the rabbit, ovulation follows the stimulus of mating. This is called *induced* ovulation; in the rabbit it occurs about ten hours after copulation due to reflex release of LH.

Table I Ovulation and Gestation Period in some Common Mammals

Species	Cycle (days)	Type Ovulation	Normal gestation period
woman	28	spontaneous	*ca.* 266
bitch	*	spontaneous	58-63
rat	4-5	spontaneous	22
mouse	4	spontaneous	19
cat	15-21	induced	65
ferret	*	induced	42
rabbit	—	induced	*ca.* 30

*these animals do not show typical cycles, but periods of oestrus (heat), twice yearly for the bitch, March-August for the ferret, in absence of pregnancy. Rabbits in the wild are seasonal breeders, but do not undergo typical cycles.

In primates, which include man, reproductive activity is also cyclical, but the cycles are termed menstrual rather than oestrous. Although each of these is centred about the release of one or more ripe ova, periodic bleeding from the uterus provides a more obvious manifestation of cyclical activity. The first appearance of the shed blood and endometrial lining of the uterus *per vaginam* is taken as marking the beginning of a new menstrual cycle, although it is really the last event of the previous one.

Except during pregnancy and in certain pathological or therapeutically induced conditions, menstrual periods occur in women throughout their reproductive life. The onset of menstrual periods, the menarche, is one of the manifestations of puberty, and commonly occurs in the human female between the ages of 12 and 15 years (see p. 42). It does not, however, necessarily mark either the onset of *regular* menstrual cycles or of full reproductive activity, and early cycles are often not associated with ovulation. Once cycles are established, they normally continue, in the absence of pregnancy, until the menopause. This, which marks the end of reproductive activity, usually occurs when the individual is in her later forties; like the menarche it is not a sudden event, but may extend over several years, as ovarian function gradually fails. After the menopause the hormonal milieu of the body has significantly changed, largely due to the disappearance of typical ovarian secretory cycles.

Among the chief characteristics of reproductive cycles in the human are:
1. menstrual bleeding, which is usually taken as marking the beginning of a cycle;

2. a more or less regular succession (pregnancy apart) of one cycle after another;
3. the occurrence of ovulation spontaneously at about mid-cycle;
4. a lack of strongly marked changes in libido throughout the cycle;
5. a lack of marked seasonal variation in fertility.

Qualifications to some of these statements will be discussed later in the text.

FEMALE REPRODUCTIVE ORGANS

Ovaries

The human ovaries during the reproductive period are flattened oval bodies, measuring up to about 3½ by 1½ by 1 cm. They lie against the wall of the true pelvis, lateral to the uterus, suspended from a backward extension of the broad ligament of the uterus which forms the suspensory mesovarium. In multiparous women the ovary usually lies with its long axis more or less vertical; its upper lateral, superior and medial borders are closely related to the Fallopian tube (oviduct) which lies in the upper border of the broad ligament (Fig. 8).

Each ovary consists of a central medulla made up of connective tissue and large convoluted blood vessels and a surrounding cortex. Except at its attachment to the broad ligament, the hilum, each organ is covered by a single layer of flattened epithelium which lies on a layer of dense connective tissue, the tunica albuginea. The term "germinal" is still applied to the cellular layer, since it used to be considered the source of the germ cells in both embryonic and post-natal life, a theory which is now largely discounted. Beneath the tunica in the cortex are large numbers (some hundreds of thousands in young women) of primordial follicles, together with follicles in varying stages of development (see below). Between the follicles lie spindle-shaped cells and connective tissue fibres. In the ovaries of many species of mammal, including some rodents and carnivores, these cells are differentiated into large polyhedral or globular elements containing lipid, which are called interstitial cells. These become larger and more prominent during pregnancy and at certain phases of the oestrous cycle, although in some species their development is greater in anoestrus, in others during pro-oestrus and oestrus. In other species, including women and other primates, interstitial cells are relatively inconspicuous. They have been associated with the secretion of both oestrogens and androgens.

In the human ovary another type of cell is found associated with vessels and nerves as they enter the ovary. These are the "hilus" cells, which resemble testicular interstitial (Leydig) cells in appearance. Hyperplasia and tumours of these cells are associated with masculinisation, and they are thought to secrete androgen.

In some species, including amphibia and some reptiles, oogenesis continues throughout the reproductive span; but in most if not all mammals and in

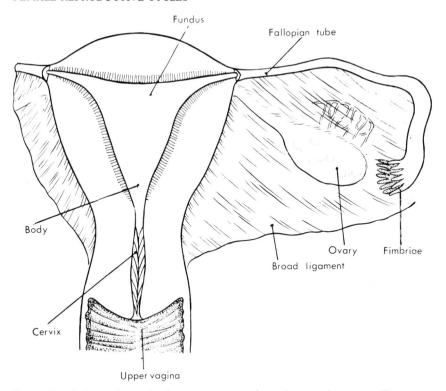

Fig. 8. Female internal reproductive organs as seen from the posterior aspect. The ovary, attached to the broad ligament is closely associated with the fimbriae of the Fallopian tube. This runs medially to join the uterus, shown in section, which can be divided into the body, fundus, and cervix through which it communicates with the vagina.

women the process is completed very early in life. In human ovaries the total population of oocytes increases during fetal life to a peak of about 6,800,000 by the fifth month, and after this declines. At birth there are about 1,000,000 normal follicles, but only some 300,000 at seven years of age. Of these only about 400 will undergo the full range of changes culminating in the shedding of a ripe ovum from the ovary at ovulation, although many more will develop to a variable but incomplete extent before undergoing the degenerative process called atresia.

The primordial follicles each contain a primary oocyte surrounded by a single layer of follicular or granulosa cells. The changes leading from a primordial follicle to a mature one take place in two stages (Fig. 9). Firstly, a primary follicle develops. This is recognised by enlargement of the oocyte, which develops a thin refractile layer around its periphery, the zona pellucida. The surrounding follicular cells enlarge and multiply to form a stratified epithelium. As these changes take place, the stromal tissue surrounding the follicle differentiates into a vascular inner layer, the theca interna, made up of secretory cells, and an outer theca externa made up largely of vascular connective tissue. As its size increases the follicle comes to lie deeper to the ovarian cortex.

The growing follicles assumes an oval shape and the ovum comes to lie eccentrically within the mass of follicular cells. When the follicle has reached about 200 μm in diameter follicular cells in the region away from the ovum begin to break down and a number of small fluid-filled spaces are formed. These coalesce to form a single cavity, the antrum, which marks the stage of a secondary follicle. Growth continues until the follicle consists of a fluid filled cyst lined by follicular cells, the ovum surrounded by these lying to one side, separated by a thin layer of cells from the fluid and attached by the basal cells to the outer wall of the follicle.

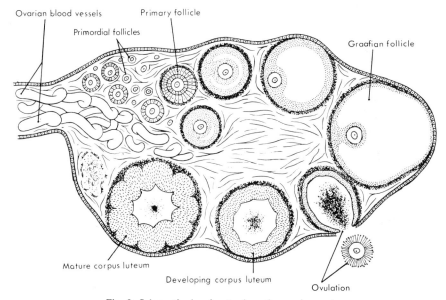

Fig. 9. Schematic drawing to show the ovarian cycle.

As it approaches maturity, the distended follicle bulges at the surface of the ovary. More spaces develop in the remaining follicular cells so that the attachment of the ovum and its cellular covering becomes loose. Changes in the surrounding tissues accompany those of follicular maturation and by the time maturity is achieved the theca interna has become a well developed and vascular sheath. Usually in the human ovary only one follicle in each cycle develops to that state of maturity which ends in rupture and ovulation, although two, three or even more ova may on occasion be released which, if fertilised, may result in multiple pregnancy.

At ovulation the oocyte together with some associated granulosa cells and follicular fluid is released from the ovary. The ruptured follicle then undergoes changes which result in the formation of a corpus luteum, which acts as an ovarian endocrine gland secreting progesterone. The walls of the follicle collapse to form a folded mass of cells usually enclosing a central mass of debris. The cells of the granulosa, together with those of the theca interna, enlarge and accumulate droplets of yellowish lipid in their cytoplasm, becoming transformed into large spherical or polygonal lutein cells. The outer ones, derived from the theca, are somewhat smaller and darker staining than the inner ones which are derived from the granulosa. Ultrastructurally lutein cells show many mitochondria and a prominent Golgi zone, together with the abundant smooth endoplasmic reticulum found in steroid secreting cells. Occasional small canaliculi bounded by microvilli occur between cells. The rich vascular supply necessary for endocrine activity develops by the ingrowth of capillaries from the theca externa into the mass of cells.

If ovulation is not followed by fertilisation and pregnancy, the corpus luteum soon begins to degenerate and is transformed to a pale scar, or corpus albicans, which disappears quite rapidly over the next cycle or so. Fertilisation and implantation of a fertilised ovum however ensures that the corpus luteum persists as a "corpus luteum of pregnancy" (see p. 53).

Most primordial ovarian follicles will never mature to the stage of ovulation. They undergo the process of degeneration called atresia, which may occur in primordial follicles or at any stage in the development of primary and secondary follicles. Vascular connective tissue extends among the granulosa cells and the theca interna hypertrophies; the granulosa cells break down and are resorbed and the ovum degenerates. Commonly the basement lamina increases in size to form a thick hyaline "glassy membrane". After a period of apparent development, the theca cells in turn are infiltrated by blood vessels and connective tissue and eventually a pale scar results which in time disappears.

Non-mammalian vertebrates show wide variations in ovarian structure and function. In viviparous fishes the ovaries provide protection and nourishment for the developing young. Some do not ovulate and fertilisation and subsequent development takes place within the ovarian follicles. Others are ovoviviparous and the eggs are retained with enough yolk to carry the embryo through its development. Structures resembling corpora lutea occur in widely divergent types of fish and in viviparous species persist during pregnancy, although they do not necessarily act as endocrine organs.

In amphibia the eggs surrounded by follicular cells bulge on stalks into the cavities of the hollow lobes of the ovary. Mature eggs are ovulated directly into the body cavity. The formation of corpora lutea has been described in some species.

Oestrogens have been found in fish and amphibian ovaries, and in frogs and some lizards degeneration of the oviducts follows ovariectomy.

Most species of birds have only one functional ovary. Asymmetry of the two developing gonads is apparent during embryonic development, and it is generally the left one together with its oviduct that becomes functional. This ovary differs greatly in appearance from those of mammals. The follicles are large and develop on follicular stalks, and a very large amount of yolk is formed. Unlike mammals, eggs may be released daily over prolonged periods of time

The avian ovary secretes oestrogen, progesterone (or a comparable substance) and androgen. The oestrogen stimulates growth of the oviduct and brings about changes in blood chemistry, notably a marked increase in calcium. Progesterone acts synergistically with oestrogen on the oviduct; its source is probably follicular, since no structure comparable with the mammalian corpus luteum is found in birds. Androgens may be produced by cells which resemble the interstitial (Leydig) cells in the mammalian testis.

The uterine cycle

The uterus is a muscular organ lined by mucosa, the endometrium, and mostly invested by an outer serous layer of peritoneum. It consists of a body, a rounded fundus and a cervix which projects into the vagina. The two oviducts extend laterally from the upper part of the uterus (Fig. 8, p. 25).

The monthly changes in the endometrium, which constitute the menstrual cycle, provide the most obvious signs of occurrence of reproductive cycles in women. As already noted it is customary to take the onset of the menstrual flow, which is really the end of one ovarian-uterine cycle, as marking the beginning of the next. Bleeding occurs when the greater part of the endometrium, which has become hypertrophic and oedematous in preparation for implantation of a fertilised ovum, breaks down, and a mixture of blood, cellular debris and secretion is shed over several days through the uterine cervix.

At the end of the phase of menstrual bleeding, about the fourth day after its onset, the endometrium consists only of a thin layer of cellular and vascular connective tissue lining the muscular wall of the uterus. There is no surface epithelium, since this has all been shed; but the deepest basal (fundic) parts of the endometrial glands remain, although the more superficial (and the greater) parts of these glands have been lost with the rest of the lining.

The survival of the fundic parts of the glands is most important, for these provide the source of epithelial cells which begin to grow out to form a new epithelial lining for the uterus as soon as the endometrial debris from the preceding cycle has been shed. At the same time the endometrial stroma begins to be re-formed and blood vessels grow towards the surface. This phase of repair is part of the proliferative phase of the cycle, during which growth processes predominate and lead to a reconstituted endometrium which is lined by a simple epithelium, and is made up of straight tubular glands lying in a vascular stroma. This phase is largely under the influence of ovarian oestrogen; it is also referred to as the follicular phase of the cycle, and it lasts until about the mid point, taken conventionally from the first day of menstrual bleeding.

The second part of the cycle is characterised by secretory rather than proliferative changes in the endometrium. Vascularity increases, the interglandular stroma becomes oedematous, and the glands lose their simple tubular form, becoming convoluted and distended with secretion. The secretory phase is mainly controlled by progesterone secreted by the corpus luteum and is often called the luteal phase. It gives way to the menstrual (bleeding) phase if no fertilised ovum embeds in the uterus in the latter half of the cycle.

The blood supply to the endometrium reaches it through branches of the uterine arteries. These ascend between the layers of the broad ligament on the lateral sides of the uterus, and anastomose with the ovarian-tubal vessels. Branches from the uterine arteries penetrate the wall of the uterus and in the vascular layer of the myometrium arcuate arteries run circumferentially towards the midline, where vessels from each side anastomose. Branches from these arcuate arteries extend towards the surface giving off basal branches to supply the deepest part (stratum basale) of the endometrium which is not shed at menstruation, and unbranched coiled arteries which supply the rich capillary bed of the superficial stratum functionale.

Menstruation is initiated by vascular activity. The coiled arteries which supply the superficial and greater part of the endometrium constrict, although not all at the same time. Each vessel remains constricted for some hours, then dilates again. The tissue thus deprived of its normal supply of blood has by this time undergone anoxic damage which increases with each phase of constriction. Intermittent constriction and dilatation continues for two days or so, after which the arteries close, then finally open shedding blood into the stroma. Blood and fragments of endometrium are cast off into the lumen and are passed vaginally, mingled with glandular secretions. The repair phase then begins again.

Although the most striking changes in the reproductive tract during the menstrual cycle are those occurring in the ovaries and endometrium, other parts of the tract also respond to the variations in hormonal secretions. The uterine cervix, vagina and Fallopian tubes show structural and functional modifications, largely dependent on the levels of circulating oestrogens and progesterone. These changes may have an important bearing on fertility and in recent years some have been studied for their possible significance in relation to contraception.

Uterine cervix

The lower part of the uterus differs both structurally and functionally from the body and the fundus. Inferiorly the body is continuous with the cervix at the internal os. Some authors also refer to the "isthmus" — the upper part of the cervix or, according to others, the lower part of the body, which is pulled up during early pregnancy to form the "lower uterine segment" of obstetricians. The mucous membrane of the uterus changes as the cervix is reached, either more or less abruptly. The mucosa of the cervix is about 2-3 mm thick, and contains many large branched mucus-secreting glands. This mucous membrane does not show the cyclical changes typical of the endometrium and is not shed at menstruation, but the secretory activity of the cervical glands and the viscosity of the mucus which normally fills the cervical canal varies with the blood oestrogen-progesterone ratio.

The cervical mucus forms a barrier to infection between the vagina and uterine cavity throughout the cycle. In early postmenstrual and the luteal phases it also offers a hindrance to the passage of sperm. At these times the gel-forming mucus consists of a very fine mesh with spaces of the order of 0.3 μm filled with a liquid phase. Under the influence of oestrogen, by mid-cycle the mucus has assumed a micellar structure with a distance between micelles of about 3 μm, and it can be readily traversed by sperm. A practical application of this change has been the treatment of infertile women with oestrogen for five days before anticipated ovulation in an attempt to decrease the viscosity of the mucus. A widely used method of assessing its viscoelastic properties ("Spinnbarkheit") is to measure the length of a thread which can be drawn out from a spot of mucus on a glass slide: this may be some three times longer with mucus sampled at the time of ovulation than at other times of the cycle.

It has been suggested that the intermicellar spaces form channels through the mucus which are opened and closed more or less rhythmically by thermal agitation of the micelles, propagating waves in the intermicellar fluid phase which carry sperm with the appropriate (normal) swimming rate towards the uterine cavity. Sperm which are either morphologically or "hydrodynamically" abnormal may not be selected for active transportation by this means. The assumption of such marked directional properties in the mucus at mid-cycle should facilitate the passage of sperm, while their absence at other phases may inhibit it.

Vagina

The changes which take place in human vaginal mucosa during the menstrual cycle are much less extensive than those in the endometrium and, indeed, in some standard texts, they tend to be dismissed somewhat summarily. In non-primates well defined cytological changes are associated with the different phases of the oestrous cycle, and the examination of the types of cell in stained vaginal smears gives a good indication of the stage reached. This correlation of cytology with the stage of the cycle is particularly clear in such mammals as the rat and guinea-pig. In these, hypertrophy of the mucosa occurs in the pre-ovulatory pro-oestrous phase, and by the time of oestrus or ovulation the superficial layers of cells have become keratinized.

In metoestrus the epithelium thins again and is invaded by large numbers of polymorphonuclear leucocytes, many of which pass into the vaginal lumen with shed epithelial cells. During dioestrus when the corpora lutea involute the vaginal epithelium remains thin and some polymorphonuclear leucocytes persist in the superficial layers. Thus vaginal smears during pro-oestrus contain nucleated epithelial cells; numerous cornified squamous cells denote oestrus; metoestrus is characterised by a few cornified cells and numerous leucocytes, and the latter type of cell still predominates in the dioestrous smear. These histological changes occur under the influence of the ovarian hormones; cornification is predominantly due to oestrogenic influence.

In women the stratified vaginal epithelium consists of several zones of cells, not usually sharply demarcated from each other. As usual in stratified epithelia, the deepest cells lying on the lamina propria are germinal and by division provide replacements for those cells lost at the surface. The germinal cells, which are small and stain more deeply than those of the more superficial layers, together with several overlying layers of large polygonal cells, constitute the basal zone. Superficial to this lies an intermediate zone made up of cells with thick cornified walls, which is succeeded by the superficial or functional zone of less closely packed cells with thinner walls. Some of these contain nuclei which show signs of degeneration. The surface cells, which are commonly flattened and contain only nuclear remnants, are shed into the lumen of the vagina. Marked keratinization such as occurs in the stratum corneum of the skin is not normally a feature of the human vaginal lining.

Oestrogen stimulates the synthesis of glycogen by cells of the vaginal epithelium, and this is particularly marked towards the time of ovulation. The glycogen contained in the desquamated cells is broken down by bacterial action to lactic acid, which accounts for the usually low pH of the vaginal fluid. Some additional shedding of the epithelium occurs at menstruation, but this involves only the more superficial layers, which reappear during the first half of the cycle. These layers increase considerably in thickness during the luteal phase, and the cells become less cornified.

The effects of hormones on the vaginal epithelium has been studied in post-menopausal women, in whom ovarian hormones are lacking. The epithelium is much reduced in thickness and may consist of no more than a thin basal zone. If oestrogen is given it comes to resemble more closely the structure seen in the normal intermenstrual phase, and cornification progressively increases in the more superficial zone. The addition of progesterone to the oestrogen results in an increase in height of the cells, loose packing and lessened cornification, characteristic of the luteal phase of the cycle.

Despite the fact that the vaginal changes during the menstrual cycle are not so marked as those occurring in the reproductive cycles of many animals, smears do show different cytological characteristics which reflect the variations in the epithelial lining. During the menstrual phase, shed vaginal cells may be obscured by the presence of mucus, endometrial debris and blood, but leucocytes, mononuclear cells and non-cornified epithelium of vaginal origin are present. The postmenstrual phase shows many "pre-cornified" cells and some cornified ones, the latter usually amounting to less than 20% of the total. Cornified cells increase in the immediate pre-ovulatory phase. At about the time of ovulation, the vaginal fluid is clear and 50-60% of its cells are cornified with few leucocytes. After ovulation the leucocytes increase greatly in number and clumps of epithelial cells replace the formerly discrete ones. The development of these features probably gives the most accurate indication that ovulation has occurred; in the succeeding luteal phase, fewer cornified cells are present.

Fallopian tubes

The Fallopian tubes are about 10 cm in length, and consist of a muscular wall lined by mucous membrane. The most lateral part of the tube, the infundibulum, consists of a funnel shaped opening, the external os, which is surrounded by processes or fimbriae, and lies close to the ovary. This leads into the ampulla, a relatively wide part of the tube, which in turn leads into a narrower region, the isthmus. Most medially the tube passes through the wall of the uterus as the intramural segment. The lining of the tube is thrown into much-branched folds, which are particularly well developed in the more lateral parts. The epithelium is simple columnar, made up of cells with cilia which beat towards the uterine opening of the tube and non-ciliated, probably secretory, cells.

The epithelium varies with different phases of the menstrual cycle. At about the time of ovulation, it is high columnar and the ciliated and non-ciliated cells are approximately equal in height, so that the luminal border appears smooth. In the premenstrual phase and in pregnancy the epithelium is lower and projections from the apices of the non-ciliated cells extend above the level of the cilia, so that the surface appears more irregular. Hence in the predominantly oestrogenic phase of the cycle the epithelium tends to be higher and the surface smoother. Oestrogens also stimulate stromal growth, as well as increasing the secretion of fluid, ciliary activity and peristaltic contractions of the muscular layer. Some data from animal experiments indicate that progesterone exerts the opposite effect. Observations on the reaction of human Fallopian tube to a variety of hormones *in vitro* have been made and it appears that under such conditions, which are of course somewhat different from those in the body, it reacts not only to steroid hormones, but also to others such as ADH and adrenal medullary hormones; this perhaps is not surprising in view of its content of smooth muscle.

The oocyte enters the Fallopian tube almost immediately after ovulation and usually spends several days (probably about three) before passing into the uterus. At the time of ovulation, the muscle of the tubes contracts at intervals of 4-8 seconds; at other times in the cycle contractions occur at longer intervals. Fertilisation usually occurs in the lateral part of the tube, and the fertilised ovum then rapidly passes to the region of the junction of the ampulla and isthmus, where it remains for several days, during which the blastocyst is developing. The timing of entry of the blastocyst into the uterus is critical for its successful implantation and survival, and this timing appears to be controlled to some extent by the hormonal effects on tubal motility.

Thus in women cyclical changes are found in all the internal reproductive organs during the menstrual cycle, and also to a lesser extent in the breasts (see p. 69). Premenstrual mastalgia, and a feeling of fullness and tingling in the week preceding menstruation is not uncommon. A high proportion of women have some premonitory symptoms a few days before their periods, and may experience a feeling of tension, depression and irritation at that time. Premenstrual water retention, which may be associated with clinically detectable oedema, is attributed to the increased level of progesterone in the second half of the cycle. The effects of hormonal influences on the central nervous system are considered in Chapter 11.

HORMONAL CONTROL OF MENSTRUAL CYCLES

Thirty years or so ago, the control of menstrual cycles was simply explained in terms of the secretion by the anterior pituitary of two gonadotropic hormones, FSH and LH, and the sequential effects of these bringing about the secretion of two steroid hormones, oestrogen and progesterone, by the ovaries. New knowledge has revealed a much greater complexity of action at these two "levels" of control and also implicated the central nervous system. The early simplistic view, however, might serve as an introductory outline against which to consider those complexities which are now understood as well as those which are still unclear. Such a scheme is as follows.

The anterior pituitary secretes FSH from the time of menstruation. This hormone is responsible for follicular development in the ovary and also stimulates the secretion of oestrogen, which in turn induces the processes of repair and proliferation of the endometrium. The first half of the cycle is thus the follicular, oestrogenic or proliferative phase.

As the oestrogen level of the plasma rises, the negative feedback effect of this steroid on the anterior pituitary results in a fall in the secretion of FSH; it also exerts a positive feedback effect which brings about the secretion of LH. This gonadotropin acts on a suitably developed (or primed) follicle and causes ovulation and then stimulates the formation of a corpus luteum and the secretion of progesterone. Progesterone is responsible for the secretory phase of the endometrium, preparing it for the reception of a fertilised ovum. The second half of the cycle is thus the luteal, progestational or proliferative one. Should fertilisation not occur the secretion of LH ceases, possibly on account of the fall in oestrogen combined with a negative feedback effect of progesterone. The corpus luteum ceases to produce progesterone: menstruation occurs, the pituitary is no longer inhibited from secreting FSH, and another cycle begins.

The availability of methods for determining the plasma levels of hormones with considerable accuracy has now made possible a much more precise analysis of the changes which occur throughout the cycle. Several aspects of the initial simple scheme must therefore be reconsidered, in the light of the following findings which are illustrated in Fig. 10:

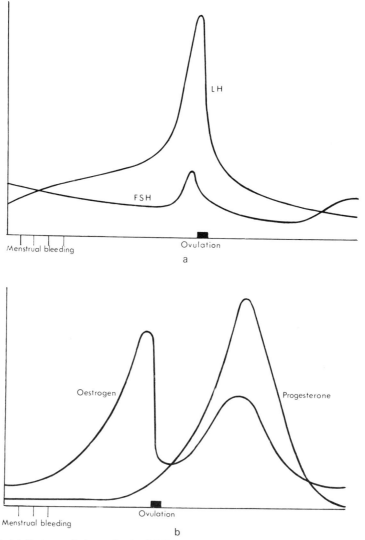

Fig. 10. (a) Patterns of plasma levels of FSH and LH in the menstrual cycle. (b) Simplified patterns of plasma levels of oestrogen and progesterone in the menstrual cycle.

1. Although the first and second halves of the cycle were commonly described as the follicular (oestrogenic) and luteal (progestational) phase respectively, both gonadotropins are in fact present in varying though appreciable amounts throughout the whole cycle; oestrogen levels are very low immediately before and during the menses and then begin to increase; the level of progesterone reaches a peak about the middle of the second half of the cycle;

2. as already described, the anterior pituitary and ovary do not form an independent endocrine complex; the pituitary is to a large extent dominated by the hypothalamus, which secretes releasing factors/hormones into the portal blood. Although at first two distinct releasing factors were postulated, each controlling the secretory activity of one of the two distinct types of cell which produce respectively FSH and LH, the evidence now available indicates that a single hormone, LH/FSH-RH, acts on both types of cell, and thus controls the secretion of both FSH and LH;

3. feedback effects, both positive and negative, are much more complex than originally postulated;

4. "local" variations in sensitivity to tropic hormones by ovarian structures and possibly utero-ovarian interactions may be of importance.

Some of these observations, at any rate, can be incorporated into a modified outline of the events underlying the menstrual cycle. Taking as the starting point the late luteal phase before the onset of menstrual bleeding, this is characterised by the beginning of growth of a number of ovarian follicles coinciding with an increase in plasma levels of FSH. The follicular growth continues through the bleeding phase of the cycle, and the level of LH also begins to rise. The latter hormone is necessary for the production of oestrogen by FSH-stimulated follicles, and under its influence the level of oestrogen also begins to increase.

The original hypothesis that two distinct hypothalmic releasing hormones controlled the secretion of the two tropic hormones FSH and LH suggested that a separate hypothalamic "centre" controlled each of the two. The acceptance that a single releasing hormone can bring about the differential secretion of the two tropic hormones necessitates some mechanism whereby the two types of secretory cell in the pars distalis respond differently. One hypothesis for which there is evidence is that the LH-secreting cells have longer latency of response to the LH/FSH-RH; local feedback effects may also play a part in this mechanism.

As oestrogen levels rise, their negative feedback effect on the secretion of FSH comes into operation, and the output of this tropic hormone by the pituitary falls; but oestrogens also exert a positive feedback effect on the secretion of LH, so that the level of LH continues to rise in the first half of the cycle. The marked rise in oestrogen during the late proliferative phase is probably a major factor in the causation of the mid-cycle peak of LH, which brings about ovulation. It has been suggested that progesterone might also play a part in the initiation of this peak, but since there is no increase in the plasma level of progesterone before the surge, this is unlikely. As shown in Fig. 10a the surge of LH is accompanied by a smaller, later starting and sooner ending rise in FSH, which may be brought about by increased progesterone.

In the post-ovulatory phase, progesterone rises to a peak and probably exerts a negative feedback effect on the secretion of LH which, after an initial sharp decline from peak value, continues to fall slowly until menstruation.

Both positive and negative feedback effects can be demonstrated experimentally, and it seems likely that these operate simultaneously, the net effect being the result of summation. Despite the continued rise in levels of oestrogen throughout the first half of the cycle, the secretion of FSH is not abolished but follows a curve, the slope of whose fall is less steep than the slope of the rise for oestrogen. This seems to be because the sensitivity of the hypothalamus to the negative feedback varies with the level of circulating oestrogen. At low levels of oestrogen, a small increase exerts a strong feedback effect, but at higher levels the feedback effect is much smaller.

Corpus luteum

If pregnancy is established the corpus luteum (of pregnancy) remains active for a considerable time (see p. 53). By contrast the life of a corpus luteum of menstruation (or ovulation), one formed in a cycle which ends in menstrual bleeding, is short. It reaches maturity in about eight days and rapidly involutes a few days later. As it does so its output of progesterone rapidly declines, and the total secretion of ovarian steroids reaches its lowest level, insufficient to maintain the endometrium, just before menstruation.

Observations on hypophysectomised women indicate that LH is necessary for continued luteal function. Some studies have been based on the use of human chorionic gonadotropin; although this substance is not identical to LH as regards its effect on the corpus luteum, probably due to its longer half-life, it is a hormone with actions similar to LH, and anti-HCG serum cross reacts with LH. Administration of such serum to monkeys had the effect of blocking ovulation if given on days 10-13 of the cycle, and of inducing early menstrual bleeding if given within a few days after ovulation. The latter observation suggests that the inactivation of LH which was produced by the serum was followed by a failure of the corpus luteum, a consequent fall in the level of circulating progesterone and endometrial breakdown. When HCG was given to women during the luteal phase of the cycle, this phase was prolonged.

In women and monkeys it thus seems that LH (or HCG) is luteotropic. In some non-primate species another tropic factor is involved, namely LTH (prolactin), which has been shown to exercise a luteotropic effect. There is no firm evidence that LTH acts in this way in women.

In some species the uterus plays a part in the control of the life span of the corpus luteum, and it has been shown that endometrium produces a luteolytic substance which, released at the end of an oestrous cycle, might destroy the cells of the corpus luteum. Prostaglandins may be involved (see p. 126). Hysterectomy in women however does not appear to change the life span of the corpus luteum, which in the absence of pregnancy seems to be predominantly under the control of LH.

Single ovulation

In women, unlike many mammals, it is usual for only a single follicle to develop to the stage at which it responds to the LH surge by ovulation, although earlier in the cycle a number of follicles begin to develop under the influence of FSH. Probably only one follicle (occasionally more) has reached the optimal stage of development to respond maximally to the appropriate balance of tropic hormones at the critical time of the cycle. As a follicle matures, it becomes more sensitive to gonadotropin, so that one slightly more advanced than the others would be more responsive to tropic hormones. Furthermore, the presence of oestrogen locally potentiates the effect of gonadotropins, so that a follicle which has grown ahead of the others and is thus secreting more oestrogen will in turn be more sensitive in its response to the gonadotropic hormones. The effect of administration of gonadotropins ("fertility drugs") is, not uncommonly, to bring about maturation of a number of follicles to the stage of ovulation, and multiple pregnancy may then result.

THE HYPOTHALAMUS AND REPRODUCTIVE CYCLES

The most distinctive difference between female and male reproductive activity, both in animals and in humans, is the cyclical activity which has been described above. The cyclical changes in structure and function of those parts of the reproductive tract responsible for the transport of the ovum, the passage of spermatozoa to the site of fertilisation and the transfer of the fertilised ovum into the uterus where it implants and thus initiates pregnancy, are largely dependent on the cyclical changes in the secretion of the ovarian hormones. Ovarian activity is not inherently cyclical, but controlled by the gonadotropic hormones of the anterior pituitary, which is largely dominated by the hypothalamus.

It is the hypothalamus itself, not the pituitary gland, which is the key to cyclical reproductive activity. This has been shown experimentally by exchanging pituitaries between male and female rats. The gland of a male animal, if transplanted beneath the median eminence of a hypophysectomised female and acquiring a "portal" blood supply, will secrete gonadotropins in the female cyclical pattern. The gland from a female showing a normal oestrous pattern similarly transplanted into a hypophysectomised male ceases to secrete cyclically and produces gonadotropins at the more or less steady rate typical of male rats.

Attempts to localise the region of the hypothalamus most closely concerned with the regulation of gonadotropic activity have made use of several experimental techniques. One of these involves the implanting of small pieces of anterior pituitary tissue directly into the substance of the hypothalamus. In areas containing releasing hormone, such implants maintain their typical cytological appearance and also secrete tropic hormones. Implants into areas containing no releasing hormone show loss of normal cytological character- istics and absence of hormone production. By this means maps have been produced indicating those regions of the hypothalamus which are capable of sustaining the normal characteristics of the implants. These "hypophysiotropic" areas have been established for several of the pituitary hormones (mostly in rats). They indicate that the releasing factors/hormones are localised to a limited region of the median basal hypothalamus although it does not necessarily follow that this is the site of their synthesis.

The site of feedback action has been studied by the implantation of small amounts of gonadal steroids into various hypothalamic areas. Oestrogen implanted into the tuber cinereum prevents the rise in plasma LH which normally follows ovariectomy, as indeed does the systemic injection of oestrogen. The hypothalamus lying anterior to the median basal region however appears to be responsive to a fall in oestrogen. Oestrogen implanted into the median eminence can exert a positive feedback effect and induce an increase in the output of LH from the pituitary but this effect is not observed if the implant is made into the pituitary itself.

Thus within a small area of the hypothalamus are situated neurons which can react to gonadal steroids in both positive and negative ways, increasing or decreasing the output of LH/FSH-RH into the portal blood.

Important as the hypothalamus is for the control of the anterior pituitary, it cannot be considered to act, except in a fairly limited way, in isolation from other parts of the nervous system. It receives a large tract of fibres, the fornix, from the hippocampal formation, as well as fibres from the sub- thalamus and frontal cortex and from secondary gustatory, olfactory and general sensory tracts. Connections from visual pathways have been described and even a direct retino-hypothalamic pathway, although the existence of this was not generally accepted until recently. Fibres arising from cells in the mammillary nuclei of the posterior hypothalamus form the first part of a hypothalamo-anterior thalamic-cingulate cortical pathway, and there are connections with the autonomic centres of the brain stem and spinal cord. Lesions of extra-hypothalamic parts of the central nervous system can influence hypothalamic-pituitary activity, and certain drugs and hormones, including "sex" steroids, become localised to parts of the central nervous system known to have hypothalamic connections and can modify its activity.

Attempts to determine how much autonomy is vested in the median basal hypothalamus, and how much of its activity is a consequence of its role as a "final common path" for influences coming from other parts of the nervous system have involved the partial or complete isolation of the median basal hypothalamus from outside neural connections by cutting around the area with a specially designed knife. Total neural isolation (deafferentation) of the median basal hypothalamus is followed by loss of cyclical activity in females, although gonadotropic secretion does not disappear; in male animals, testicular function continues. The medial basal hypothalamus can apparently produce, release and regulate the various releasing factors in the absence of afferent neural connections; but a cyclical pattern of release of LH/FSH-RH appears to be dependent on the influence of areas of the nervous system lying outside the median basal hypothalamic zone.

Direct transfer of the details of these findings to humans cannot be assumed. Nevertheless it is clear that the hypothalamo-pituitary-ovarian system is the central "axis" concerned in the control of menstrual as well as oestrous cycles, and that disturbances of the former can result from a malfunction at any of the "levels" involved in this control. This is considered further on p. 104.

Disorders of menstruation

The commonest cause of menstrual disturbance that the student will encounter is pregnancy. Conversely, widespread use of oral contraceptives has given prominence to the symptom of post-pill amenorrhoea. At each end of reproductive life are the problems of delayed menarche and those of the menopause, mostly resolved by the passage of time and the understanding of a sympathetic physician. However, the concept of the use of hormones at the time of the menopause and into later years is still hotly debated. Beyond these everyday examples stretches a long list of disorders, well listed in most textbooks of endocrinology.

Briefly, it is customary to distinguish primary amenorrhoea, a situation in which a female has never menstruated, from secondary amenorrhoea which is a failure of established function. In each case there may be:

    a. gonadal causes
    b. hypothalamo—pituitary causes
    c. extrinsic causes (other endocrine or metabolic disorders).

Table II gives examples.

Hormone-secreting tumours, particularly of ovarian origin, may also give rise to disturbances of menstrual cycles. Arrhenoblastomas constitute one type of these. Structurally they may show tubules resembling testicular tissue and a variable degree of development of interstitial type cells; about 25% are malignant. They are associated with severe masculinisation, hirsutism, enlargement of the clitoris, shrinkage of the breasts, assumption of male type of bodily contour and amenorrhoea. Other types include granulosa cell tumours, thecomas and luteomas, which may on occasion be associated with virilisation. Hilus cell tumours have already been noted (see p. 24).

Hirsutism

Excessive development of hair in the female is known as hirsutism. The extra hair growth is commonly seen on the upper lip, the sides of face and chin and in the general body hair. It is also evident between the breasts, around the areolae, and shows a male distribution on the abdomen. In isolation, hirsutism may be a minor disability, but, together with virilism, it must be considered abnormal. Stigmata of virilism include thinning of the hair of the scalp, temporal hair recession, deepening of the voice, hypertrophy of muscle, acne, clitoromegaly and either oligomenorrhoea or amenorrhoea. When virilism accompanies hirsutism, increased androgen secretion is the rule.

Most commonly seen is idiopathic hirsutism and this ranges from a mild increase in body hair to a major endocrine upset. Nevertheless, it is important to consider other causes such as constitutional and racial, physiological (menopausal) imbalance and iatrogenic origin. More serious are

Table II

	Primary amenorrhoea	Secondary amenorrhoea
Gonadal	chromosomal abnormalities (e.g. Turner's Syndrome) congenital hypoplasia	tumours (non-masculinising) tumours (masculinising) polycystic ovaries (Stein-Leventhal Syndrome)
	tumours (non-masculinising) tumours (masculinising) agenesis, gynaetresia (absence of uterus and vagina)	
Hypothalamico-pituitary	tumours vascular lesions and infections	as for Primary with inappropriate lactation (galactorrhoea)
Extrinsic	congenital adrenal hyperplasia	Cushing's syndrome Addison's disease Thyroid disease Inanition, malabsorption, anorexia nervosa Diabetes mellitus

ovarian factors such as polycystic disease and tumours, as well as adreno-cortical lesions such as Cushing's syndrome and congenital adrenal hyperplasia.

The vast majority of cases of idiopathic hirsutism encompass a minor but unpleasant disability without menstrual disturbance. Even so, there is usually a small elevation in plasma testosterone. Treatment may be directed towards adrenocortical or ovarian androgen suppression, but this is rarely successful. Depilatory waxes and creams are available and electrolysis is often resorted to. The simple method of shaving is generally effective but unaesthetic. Where plasma androgens are considerably raised or menstruation is affected, further investigation and attempts at treatment are justified. Rarer causes are: pituitary tumours (acromegaly), gonadal maldevelopment, ovarian agenesis, inter-sex states, anorexia nervosa and porphyria.

4

Puberty

"Puberty", wrote F. H. A. Marshall in 1922, "or the period at which the organism becomes sexually mature, is marked by the occurrence of those constitutional changes whereby the two sexes become fully differentiated. It is at this period that the secondary organs of reproduction undergo a great increase in size...."

Despite the sometimes imprecise use of the term, the achievement of puberty implies that an individual has become functionally capable of procreation. Adolescence, which is sometimes referred to as if it were synonymous with puberty, signifies the period of growth between childhood and maturity, ending with cessation of somatic growth. Epiphysial fusion, which irrevocably marks the end of growth, is not usually completed until some years after puberty.

PHYSICAL CHANGES

The maturation of the reproductive organs which leads up to puberty is accompanied by external signs which indicate its progress, usually extending over several years. In girls development of the breasts and in boys growth of the external genital organs occurs; in both sexual hair develops. The progress of puberty has been classified by stages. The first sign of breast development in girls after the pre-adolescent elevation of the nipple is budding (that is elevation of the nipple and breast as a small mound), widening of the areola and its elevation on sub-areolar tissue, commonly begins just after 11 years of age, and development of the breasts continues for about four years. Pubic hair usually appears about half a year after the beginning of changes in the breast and reaches adult type, quantity and distribution before breast development is complete, at an average age of 14½ years. The first menstrual period, the menarche, in a series of girls studied in this country was found to occur at 13½ years, that is before the changes in breasts and development of sexual hair are complete.

In boys some growth of the testicles takes place between 6 and 10 years. Marked testicular enlargement and pigmentation and thinning of the scrotal skin begin at a mean age of just over 11½ years, followed a year later by penile growth; the adult size and form of the genitals is achieved at just under 15 years of age. Growth of coarse and curly hair begins at a mean age of 13½ years, and continues to about 15 years, although extension of hair up the anterior abdominal wall and full development of facial hair often does not occur until the twenties.

Puberty in both sexes is associated with an increased rate of growth commonly referred to as the adolescent growth spurt. During this spurt sexual differentiation of the skeleton occurs, girls developing the typical female pelvis, boys showing growth of the shoulder girdle. Many children put on fat just before the growth spurt. During this period boys usually show a decrease in the amount of fat in the limbs, while in girls it increases in the regions of the breasts and pelvis. In girls the peak rate of increase in height usually occurs at just over 12 years of age, when the changes in the breasts and growth of pubic hair are at a relatively early stage. In boys the peak of growth is at about 14 years, significantly later in terms of both chronological age and of the degree of sexual maturation, and at this time growth of the larynx leads to "breaking" of the voice. The facial appearance changes as the air sinuses within the facial bones increase their size. The growth of the maxillary sinuses is largely associated with the eruption of the permanent teeth, which except for the third molars takes place in the pre-pubertal period. During puberty however the frontal sinuses extend into the frontal bone above the orbits, and increased formation of bone occurs in the brow ridges so that the length of the skull increases.

The age of onset of pubertal changes and their rate of progress varies appreciably in individual girls and boys. Furthermore, surveys in countries other than Britain have produced figures which differ somewhat from those quoted; this is hardly surprising, since factors which may influence the time of onset and rate of progress of pubertal changes vary considerably between different populations. It has also been proposed that sexual maturation is associated with a critical body weight, which must be attained for pubertal changes to occur. Since both skeletal growth and total body weight are dependent on adequate nutrition, improved nutrition might well be a factor in the observed decrease in menarchial age. Supporting evidence for a nutritional influence comes from observations that sexual maturity tends to be reached earlier, in both girls and boys, in those with a greater body weight and skeletal maturity.

HORMONAL CHANGES

Complex hormonal changes take place before and during puberty. A major factor is an alteration of the activity of the hypothalamic-anterior pituitary-gonadal axis, from which follow the changes in the reproductive organs and the external signs of growth of sexual hair and of the breasts. An increase in the secretion of pituitary gonadotropins stimulates growth and maturation of the ovaries and testes to the stage at which they can produce mature ova and spermatozoa, and also brings about increased secretion of gonadal steroids. It is the latter hormones which effect the external signs associated with puberty. The increased output of these hormones occurs before the full maturation of germ cells, and early menstrual cycles are commonly anovulatory. The adrenal cortex plays a part in the pubertal changes, secreting androgens which stimulate the growth of pubic and axillary hair in children of both sexes.

The hormonal changes associated with sexual maturation have been established by studies using a variety of methods for the assay of gonadotropic and gonadal hormones during childhood and at various phases of puberty. Precise comparison of the findings of different authors is difficult because of differences in the groups examined and in techniques used for assay of hormones. Among the variables are the age of the individuals studied, the kind of sample taken (urine or blood), the type of assay used (bio-assay or immuno-assay), and whether or not serial assays were made for individual subjects. Some methods of assay are not as reliable as others, and hormone levels are known to fluctuate from day to day and even from one time of day to another in any 24-hour period.

The changes of endocrine activity underlying the onset of puberty do not depend on the development by the adenohypophysis of the ability to secrete the gonadotropic hormones, since the gland is capable of such secretion from an early stage. The fetal pituitary can secrete FSH and LH by about the third month *in utero,* and the administration of LH/FSH-RH to an infant of five weeks has been shown to result in a rise in plasma LH. LH/FSH-RH is present in the immature hypothalamus, and both gonadotropins are present in the plasma and are excreted in the urine during early childhood. The amounts excreted increase as childhood progresses and particularly just before or during the development of puberty. Compared with pre-pubertal children total urinary excretion in adults is some twelvefold greater for LH and sixfold for FSH, and the plasma concentrations show an increase of 2 - 3 fold in both sexes.

In girls, puberty is associated with increased secretory activity of both the ovaries and the adrenal cortex. Oestrogens secreted under the stimulus of the increased amounts of FSH stimulate growth of the endometrium and muscular wall of the uterus and of the vagina. The plasma levels of oestrogens and their urinary secretion increase as sexual maturation proceeds. Androgens, which are present in the urine of girls from early childhood, also increase, and stimulate the growth of pubic and axillary hair. The adrenal cortex secretes oestrone and some progesterone in the pre-pubertal phase; when ovulation begins, the corpus luteum is the major source of this latter hormone. The secretion of LH, as well as that of FSH, increases during puberty, the increase of the former hormone in mid-puberty probably occurring in response to the stimulus of oestrogen. Before the development of this response, the LH surge required for ovulation is lacking, and the early anovulatory cycles will not be accompanied by the formation of corpora lutea.

The physical changes of puberty in boys are mainly due to the increased secretion of testicular androgens, which stimulate growth of the penis, scrotum and of pubic, axillary and body hair. Androgens also increase the rate of growth, so that height increases rapidly. The major source is the interstitial Leydig cells of the testes, which respond to the increased secretion of LH(ICSH) by the pituitary. This hormone is detectable in the urine of young boys, but increases markedly in amount from about nine years of age through to the late teens, with a particularly marked rise in the three years leading into puberty. As already noted the adrenal cortex contributes some androgens. The testes also secrete oestrogens and their urinary excretion increases as maturation proceeds; the adrenal cortex may contribute to these and some may be formed by conversion from androgens. FSH appears to play a more restricted role in pubertal changes in boys. Its influence on spermatogenesis gives it an important role in the development of fertility, probably by increasing the binding of testosterone by the seminiferous tubules. This maintains a high level of testosterone in the testes, which is probably important in the initiation of spermatogenesis.

It might be assumed that the secretion of androgens by the adrenal cortex occurs under the influence of a pituitary hormone. Adrenal cortical activity is indeed largely under the control of ACTH; but the latter does not normally stimulate the secretion of large amounts of androgenic steroids, although it may do so in pathological states such as the adrenogenital syndrome (see p. 90). If ACTH is the factor concerned in the increased output of androgenic steroids in the pubertal period (particularly in girls) then the adrenal cortex of pubertal girls responds to the tropic hormone in a way different from that of mature individuals.

CAUSAL FACTORS

The age onset of puberty and the time for the completion of pubertal changes varies from one individual to another. Studies of groups of children however have enabled the derivation of mean ages for given populations and the degrees of deviation from the mean. Menarche, which offers a readily determinable point in pubertal development, although not in itself necessarily indicative of sexual maturity, has often been taken as a convenient "marker" in studies of puberty in girls.

In parts of the world such as Western Europe and the U.S.A. for which reliable records are available the age at menarche had decreased steadily since about the middle of the last century by as much as four months per decade. A variety of factors might have contributed to this, among them improved public health and nutrition. Reference has been made already to the association with puberty of an increased rate of growth in height, and studies have shown that "peak height velocity" usually reaches a maximum during early puberty and, in girls, before menarche.

Climatic factors have also been suggested as influences affecting the age of onset of puberty, and some authors consider that puberty takes place earlier in tropical than in temperate climates. One study recorded the age of menarche in two series of Nigerian girls, and found that it occurred some six months later than in English girls. Pubertal changes in Nigerian boys however occurred at about the same age as in English boys, although the onset of the various phases cannot be timed as precisely as the single event of the first menstrual bleeding.

Even if climate does affect the onset and progress of puberty, a number of factors have to be taken into account: notably, physical activity; environmental factors such as temperature and daylight to darkness ratios with their great variation between tropical, temperate, and arctic latitudes. But adaptation of the population, by creating the artificial environments of heated houses and by varying their clothing, may profoundly modify the influence of basic environmental factors on functions of the body. Results of experiments using animals, such as a series which showed that exposure to cold influenced the onset of puberty in rats (indicated by the time of vaginal opening) cannot readily be applied to man. Diet and the level of nutrition which influence growth and development also vary greatly in different populations. Light is known to exert a powerful modulating influence on the timing of reproductive cycles in many animals and there is some evidence that it has an effect on man. The observation that blind girls reach menarche earlier than those with normal light perception might suggest some effect mediated possibly via the pineal body (see p. 133). Genetic influences may also operate and studies have shown, for example, that the age at menarche differs significantly less between identical than between non-identical twins. Racial genetic factors are probably not so influential, and many apparently "racial" differences in age of puberty are probably due to environmental influences.

Precocious Puberty

Abnormally early development of pubertal changes may be due to a variety of causes, all of which lead to a premature and abnormal increase in the production of steroid sex hormones. Distinction has been made between true and apparent precocious puberty, the former being the premature development of activity in an otherwise normal hypothalamo-pituitary-gonadal system, the latter associated with a pathological condition. A further distinction can be made between isosexual precocious puberty, when the premature development is consistent with the sex of the individual, and heterosexual precocity when there is precocious development of secondary sexual characteristics of the opposite sex.

So called "idiopathic" sexual precocity occurs with no detectable lesion of the central nervous system, pituitary or gonads, although it may be that the lesion is so small as to be undetected. However, a variety of intracranial lesions may be associated with precocity, such as tumours in or adjacent to the hypothalamus, as well as disorders such as hydrocephalus and post-encephalitic conditions. Signs of sexual precocity may appear at any time after birth, with as many as 20% of girls with this condition menstruating by 2½ years of age. As well as this early onset, the cycles may be typical ovulatory ones, and a number of early pregnancies have been reported, with one girl delivering a normal infant at an age of 5 years 7 months. A premature growth spurt occurs in these children, but it is followed by retardation and early cessation of growth.

Precocious puberty may be associated, although uncommonly, with ovarian neoplasms. In such instances, the effects are those of a primary excess of steroid hormones, not an activation of the hypothalamo-pituitary axis. By contrast, a primary excess of androgenic steroids, as in congenital virilizing adrenal hyperplasia (see p. 90) or adrenal cortical tumours, can induce heterosexual precocity in girls, with growth of pubic and facial hair, voice changes and enlargement of the clitoris. In boys early excess of androgens may produce precocious isosexual development, although in both sexes pubic hair may develop early without precocious sexual maturation.

Hypothalamus and puberty

The association of certain lesions of the central nervous system with precocious puberty in humans indicates that a neural influence may be involved in the timing of normal pubertal changes. Indeed, considering what is now known about hypothalamic control of the function of the anterior pituitary, it would be surprising if this were not so. Experiments on animals have reinforced this view, and it seems likely that the key to the onset of puberty may be a change in sensitivity of some part of the hypothalamus to the feedback effect of gonadal hormones. The negative feedback effect of hormones secreted by the mature gonads applies also in immaturity, and removal of one testis or ovary is followed by the enlargement of the remaining one under the influence of an increased output of pituitary gonadotropin. Castration of immature rats results in an increased secretion of FSH, and a comparable effect is found in children with failure of gonadal development and consequent diminished secretion. Administration of testosterone or oestrogens inhibits the output of gonadotropins from the pituitary in such subjects, but the amount needed to bring about this inhibition is far smaller than that required to exert a similar effect in mature subjects.

These and other observations have led to the formulation of the hypothesis that the onset of puberty is associated with a decreased sensitivity of some neural 'centre' to the inhibitory (negative) feedback effect of gonadal hormones. In the pre-pubertal years, the small amounts of these hormones circulating in the blood are sufficient to suppress the activity of those parts of the central nervous system responsible for the synthesis and/or release of LH/FSH-RH. At the appropriate time the neural structures become less sensitive to such negative feedback, secretion of the releasing hormone is no longer suppressed, and as a result the pituitary secretes gonadotropins. The gonads are capable of responding to the stimulus of these by producing steroids, which in turn bring about the physical changes of puberty and act as an effective feedback mechanism only when their re-set threshold level is reached.

The hypothalamus is certainly involved in this process, although it is unlikely to be the only part of the central nervous system concerned, since other areas are known to influence endocrine activity, acting via the hypothalamus which serves as a "final common path" to the adenohypophysis. The pituitary itself may play a part by exhibiting, for example, a low sensitivity to LH/FSH-RH in the early years of life, and an increasing sensitivity as puberty approaches. In this event, the output of gonadotropins would increase towards puberty even if there were no increased secretion of the releasing hormone into the portal blood.

In summary, our present understanding of the factors underlying puberty is extensive but far from complete. The hormonal changes bringing about growth of the gonads and secretion of gonadal hormones and the secondary effects of the latter on growth and maturation are reasonably clear, but further studies using sensitive assay techniques for hormones in plasma are desirable. The role of the hypothalamus is appreciated; but the detailed interrelationships between it and the rest of the nervous system in relation to the onset of puberty are largely unexplained. Factors such as climate and day length, as well as nutrition and general health, seem to play some part in the timing of pubertal changes, although it is difficult to isolate single factors from the complex of environmental ones.

5

Pregnancy, Parturition and Lactation

Initiation of pregnancy

Oocytes normally enter the oviducts almost immediately after ovulation. Fertilisation, if it is to occur, takes place in the lateral part of the tube. Each fertilised ovum is then moved towards the uterine end, where it remains until its passage into the uterus. During this time the endometrium is increasingly under the influence of the rising titre of progesterone secreted by the corpus luteum, its stroma becoming more oedematous and the glands filling with secretion.

The first meiotic division of the oocyte is completed just before ovulation. This results in equal division of chromatin between the two daughter cells, but in an unequal division of cytoplasm. Thus one of the secondary oocytes is a larger cell than the other; the smaller, made up of a very small amount of cytoplasm and a nucleus, constitutes the first polar body which is expelled. Immediately following this the second meiotic division of the remaining oocyte begins. This proceeds only to metaphase which is the stage at which fertilisation occurs. The penetration of the oocyte by the head of the sperm is followed by completion of the second meiotic division, which again results in the formation of two unequal cells, each having an equal mass of chromatin, but one retaining most of the cytoplasm; the smaller cell forms the second polar body, which soon disappears. In the larger cell, which is now called an ovum, the nuclei of the oocyte and the sperm fuse, so that the diploid number of chromosomes (in the human, 22 pairs of autosomes plus two sex chromosomes) is restored. The time available for fertilisation of an oocyte in women is probably about 24 hours after ovulation, after which time the egg begins to degenerate.

After fertilisation the ovum, while still in the tube, undergoes a series of mitotic divisions although it does not increase in size. The result is the formation of a round mass of cells, the morula, still surrounded by the zona pellucida (see p. 25). A central cavity then develops in the morula, so that a fluid-filled cyst is formed, the blastula or blastocyst. The cells of this, called blastomeres, become arranged into an outer layer, the trophoblast, and an inner cell mass bulging into the central fluid-filled cavity; the zona pellucida has disintegrated by this stage, which is at the fourth or fifth day after ovulation, thus allowing the blastocyst to expand and flatten.

The developing fertilised human ovum probably enters the cavity of the uterus about 3½ days after ovulation, in the morula stage, and lies free for a short time. By the sixth or seventh day the process of implantation is well established although the scarcity of early human implantation sites available for study makes precise timing difficult. In macaque monkeys and cats, for example, implantation is thought to occur 10 and 14 days after fertilisation, respectively. A greater delay than usual occurs in lactating animals; rats mated at the first post-partum oestrus may show a delay in implantation up to 20 days, the time being greater with larger litters being suckled. In the wild a number of species show delayed implantation which is not associated with lactation. In the European badger an ovum fertilised in July may develop to a blastocyst which lies free in the uterus until the following January before implantation, so that the young are born in the spring. The hormonal basis for this phenomenon has been investigated experimentally, but the conclusions reached have not all been in agreement, no doubt due to some extent to the difficulty of reproducing artificially the precise hormonal pattern found in normal animals. It seems probable however that implantation is delayed in the absence of an appropriate plasma level of oestrogens in relation to the activity of the corpus luteum. In wild animals the delay may last until the resumption of appropriate pituitary gonadotropic secretion results in growth of the corpus luteum and consequent progestational development of the endometrium, which allows implantation to take place.

The first stage in implantation is presumably apposition of the trophoblast and uterine epithelium. This is followed by intimate association of the two elements, with disappearance of cell boundaries between trophoblast and uterine epithelial cells, the latter being probably phagocytosed by the former. The cells of the trophoblast then actively invade the endometrium, which responds by undergoing a hypertrophic reaction which converts it into decidua (see below). The trophoblastic cells play an active part in the nutrition of the inner cell mass, from which develops the embryo and certain associated structures such as the amnion.

The maternal hormones, which have played an essential role in the initiation of pregnancy, continue their influence once it is established. A new set of factors appears once the fetal endocrine glands have differentiated, since these are actively secretory throughout a great part of intrauterine life, and play a particularly important role in the development of the fetal reproductive system. There is also some interdependence between the fetal and maternal endocrine systems. Before the fetal glands are formed the placenta, the organ for metabolic exchange between mother and fetus, seems to be established in some species including man, as a major source of hormones. Species differences however are marked, and while the human placenta contains progesterone, that of the cow and bitch, among others, does not.

Placental development

During the process of implantation the blastocyst by a process of cellular proliferation and enzymatic digestion burrows into the hypertrophied endometrial lining of the uterus which is now known as the decidua. Proliferating trophoblast closes the small hole through which the blastocyst entered the thickness of the mucosa so that it becomes completely buried. The decidua lying between the blastocyst and the outer layers of the uterine wall is known as the decidua basalis; that overlying the blastocyst and separating it from the uterine lumen as the decidua capsularis; while that of the rest of the uterine lining is the decidua parietalis (Fig. 11).

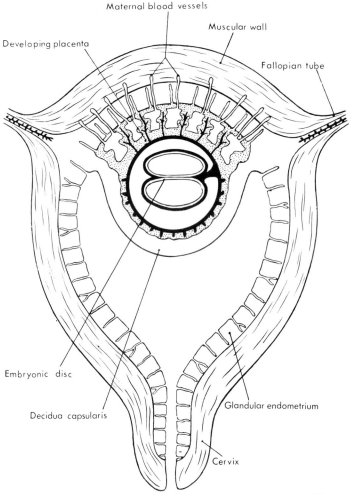

Fig. 11. Coronal section through a uterus in the early pregnant state. (Redrawn from Cunningham's "Textbook of Anatomy", 11th edition.)

The placenta is developed over the extent of the decidua basalis, and is derived from maternal (decidual) and embryonic (trophoblastic) components. After embedding in the decidua the trophoblast proliferates and differentiates into two layers, an outer one in which the cell boundaries largely break down to form a syncytium, the syncytiotrophoblast, and an inner one in which the cell structure persists, the cytotrophoblast. The cytotrophoblast is lined by extra-embryonic mesoderm, which also surrounds the embryonic tissues. Later cavitation occurs within this mesoderm, so that one layer lines the inner aspect of the cytotrophoblast and another surrounds the developing embryo; the two layers remain continuous with each other at the body stalk, in which develop the vessels linking the embryo to the placenta. The trophoblast now forms the chorionic epithelium; it continues to erode the decidua, whose cells are increasing in size and accumulating glycogen and lipid—characteristics of the decidual reaction.

The next stage in the formation of the placenta is a breakdown of areas of the still proliferating syncytiotrophoblast so that it becomes permeated with lacunae, and the erosion by the growing chorion of the walls of uterine blood vessels. This erosion results in the establishment of a flow of maternal blood through the spaces in the trophoblast, so that the chorionic tissue is bathed by maternal blood.

The fully formed human placenta is a disc-shaped structure. It consists of a chorionic plate, from which villi extend towards the decidua. Each villus consists of an outer shell of syncytiotrophoblast and an inner layer of cytotrophoblast which covers a core of connective tissue derived from the extra-embryonic mesoderm (Fig.12). These components make up the fetal part of the placenta. The layer of cytotrophoblast becomes less conspicuous as pregnancy advances and virtually disappears as term approaches. Some of the villi (anchoring) extend to the decidua and are attached to it; others simply project into the intervillous space, which is filled with maternal blood. The maternal part of the placenta is derived from the decidua basalis. After delivery of the fetus the placenta separates from the uterus and is expelled with the membranes, forming the 'after birth'.

HORMONES AND PREGNANCY

Corpus luteum and progesterone

The role of the luteal hormone, progesterone, in the establishment of pregnancy has already been partially considered. In the pre-implantation phase the uterus is prepared for implantation; the endometrial glands are stimulated to secrete and the interglandular stroma accumulates fluid. This change from a proliferative to a secretory endometrium is necessary so that the blastocyst can implant into a lining which has been appropriately conditioned. The tubal delay imposed by the action of progesterone before

Fetal blood vessel   Syncytiotrophoblast
Cytotrophobast   Extraembryonic mesoderm

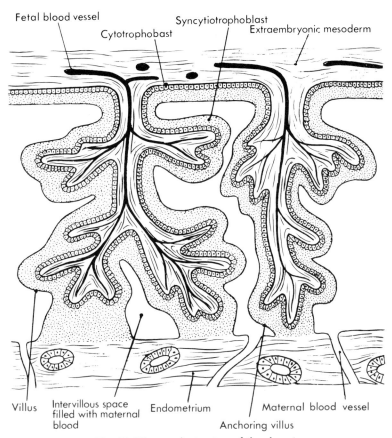

Villus   Intervillous space   Endometrium   Maternal blood vessel
filled with maternal
blood   Anchoring villus

Fig. 12. Microscopic structure of the placenta.

the ovum passes into the uterus allows the endometrium to develop beyond its 'ovulatory' state. Progesterone is essential for the initiation and for the continuance of pregnancy, and fertilisation results in the persistence of the corpus luteum (corpus luteum of pregnancy) which continues to develop and increases its secretion of this hormone. In contrast, in the later part of a cycle in which fertilisation has not occurred the corpus luteum breaks down and the plasma level of progesterone falls steeply, with resulting menstrual bleeding.

Thus, while secretory luteal tissue can normally be considered a prerequisite of pregnancy, there is considerable variation between different species of mammals in the length of time for which secretory corpora lutea are essential for its continuation without administration of exogenous hormones. These variations are correlated with the ability of the placenta to synthesise progesterone, and different species can be considered as lying at different points on a line between total dependence on the corpus luteum for the maintenance of pregnancy and tolerance of early removal of all luteal tissue, in other words placental dependency.

Although in many mammalian species the corpora lutea (for they are generally multiple) do not regress before pregnancy reaches full term, in some of these pregnancy may continue to term if ovariectomy is carried out relatively late. In some primates, although relatively few species have been studied, the ovaries with their contained corpora lutea are apparently not essential after about the first sixth of pregnancy, and the placenta soon becomes the main source of circulating progesterone. Large amounts (up to 290mg/day) of this hormone are produced by the human placenta.

Progesterone appears to be essential to the maintenance of pregnancy in all species so far studied. This is largely due to its effect on the contractile activity of the uterus, which is inhibited by appropriate amounts of the hormone. The resulting quiescence allows the retention of the blastocysts, and after implantation is essential to prevent the expulsion of the conceptus.

In species in which the maintenance of pregnancy is dependent on the continued presence of corpora lutea in the ovaries, a quantitative relationship between the number of corpora lutea, the number of fetuses and the time for which the fetuses can be retained in the uterus, has been established. Experimentally this has been done using pseudopregnant animals in which the ovaries contain corpora lutea, but there is no conceptus in the uterus. Such a condition can be easily induced in rabbits by mating females with a sterile (vasectomized) male; this results in ovulation and subsequent luteal development without pregnancy. The receptivity of the pseudopregnant uterus can then be determined by introducing blastocysts obtained from fertile matings, and observing how many are expelled and how many implant. Ovariectomy offers a means of controlling the number of corpora lutea present and their period of secretory activity.

Such studies indicate, firstly, that a minimum number of corpora lutea, probably two, is needed for any endometrial proliferation to occur, but that this minimal number is not enough to ensure retention of any appreciable number of blastocysts. Secondly, the proportion of blastocysts retained increases with the number of corpora lutea, while eight or more corpora lutea are necessary to bring about a sufficiently quiescent state of the uterus for retention of most implanted blastocysts. Ovariectomy in later pregnancy in rabbits and in rats is followed by an increase in intrauterine pressure due to muscular contraction so that the fetuses are crushed. The amount of progesterone needed for the continuance of pregnancy also depends to some extent on the uterine volume and thus on size of the litter. Pregnancy in rabbits whose ovaries have been removed can be maintained by the administration of progesterone; if this is given in less than optimal amounts, those animals with smaller litters will remain pregnant longer than those with larger ones.

Activity of the corpus luteum is dependent on pituitary LH, at any rate before chorionic gonadotropin is produced. Hypophysectomy at a critical time can cause luteal regression with effects on pregnancy comparable to those of ovariectomy.

Placenta and progesterone

In those species, including man, in which removal of the ovaries at a relatively early stage of pregnancy is not followed by expulsion of the fetuses, the placenta assumes responsibility for the synthesis of progesterone. Even in these species however the corpora lutea are actively secretory both before and after implantation, although there is a gradual shift of steroid secretion from corpus luteum to placenta. In those such as the rat in which maintenance of pregnancy depends on the corpus luteum there is some indirect evidence that the placenta can synthesise some progesterone, although not in amounts adequate to replace that from luteal tissue. Placental progesterone exerts a local effect on the myometrium of the uterus, and inhibits contraction of the muscle immediately underlying the placenta; this inhibitory effect decreases beyond the placental boundary. The mode of action of progesterone in this respect seems to be the suppression both of spontaneous electrical activity in myometrium and of the capacity of the muscle to propagate an action potential.

The concentration of progesterone is high in blood at the placental site, but despite transport of the hormone along vascular and lymphatic channels and its presence in tissue fluid, the level progressively decreases away from the placenta. The high local concentration of progesterone might account for the inability to reproduce the effects of placental progesterone and the failure to inhibit parturition in some species by administering the hormone systemically. An additional factor is that progesterone is rapidly broken down in the blood—a half-life of six minutes has been proposed—and a direct injection into the blood of the intervillous space might be the only way of reproducing the placental action. It is clear however that in those species in which ovariectomy is followed by the termination of pregnancy, progesterone reaching the uterus via the systemic circulation is essential for gestation to continue, whether or not there is any significant elaboration of the hormone by the placenta.

The production of progesterone by the placenta depends on the availability of cholesterol as the starting point of a cholesterol-pregnenolone-progesterone sequence of synthesis. Placental tissue does not synthesise a significant amount of progesterone from acetate, and little seems to be derived from available pregnenolone from extra-placental sources. The synthetic process seems to be largely independent of any regulating factors other than placental weight, and the production of progesterone increases along with placental growth, which decreases in the last few weeks of pregnancy. Throughout pregnancy the plasma levels of progesterone and the urinary levels of its excreted metabolites, notably pregnanediol, reflect the maternal synthesis of the hormone. An initial peak is due to luteal activity; this is succeeded by a brief decline, followed by a secondary peak indicative of the development of placental synthesis. In woman, the level increases gradually from the tenth week up to shortly before term, but the ovarian contribution is unimportant after the first three months.

The source of cholesterol for the placental synthesis of progesterone is largely maternal, although fetal tissues, notably the adrenals, testes and ovaries, possess the appropriate enzyme systems for the utilisation of acetate in the formation of cholesterol and of pregnenolone. Little synthesis of progesterone occurs in the fetus.

The utilisation of progesterone by the uterus has already been noted. The steroid also reaches the fetus across the placenta and various fetal tissues are able to utilise it. The fetal adrenals, for example, can convert progesterone into a variety of corticosteroids, reactions which the placenta is unable to carry out; this is further considered in Chapter 6.

Oestrogens

Oestrogens are produced in considerable quantity during pregnancy, and amounts both in blood and urine generally increase as pregnancy progresses. In the human, pregnancy urine contains oestrone, oestradiol and large amounts of oestriol. The latter oestrogen is found only in primates, notably chimpanzees, gorillas and humans. Oestrone is the predominant compound excreted in some species, such as pigs, goats, cows and horses.

Oestrogens are important for uterine growth, which involves protein synthesis and the production of enzymes necessary for muscular contraction and energy mechanisms. These steroids are produced by the ovarian follicles and in the human the corpus luteum has the requisite enzymes to synthesise them from acetate. In those species which have a long gestation period the placenta is an important source of oestrogens, while in species with a short gestation, such as the rat, the ovarian follicles remain the chief source. Placental synthesis has been demonstrated by the extraction of oestrogens from placental tissue, by the observation that blood and urinary oestrogens fall sharply after delivery of the placenta, and by studies which show that placental tissues can synthesise these compounds *in vitro*.

Androgens (C_{19}) which form the starting point for the synthesis of oestrogens can be derived from the C_{21} compounds pregnenolone and progesterone. The placenta however does not have the appropriate enzymes for such a step, and the C_{19} compounds which it utilises originate in the fetus, notably in the fetal adrenal cortex, and are then transformed to oestrogens by the placenta.

This interdependence of fetal and placental tissues for the production of oestrogens has given rise to the concept of the feto-placental unit, the fetus and the placenta both being necessary for the synthesis of compounds which neither can produce in isolation.

Protein hormones

HCG. At one time or another synthesis of a number of protein and peptide hormones has been attributed to the placenta, but claims for a placental origin of, for example, ACTH, MSH and ADH have not been sustained. As early as 1905 it was proposed that some substance arising from the placenta was associated with the persistence of the corpus luteum in early pregnancy. The notable publication by Ascheim and Zondek in 1927 reported that ovarian follicular growth and formation of corpora lutea could be stimulated in immature female mice by injecting extracts of blood or urine of pregnant women. These observations formed the basis of the Ascheim-Zondek test for pregnancy. Although it was at first thought that the active substance concerned was secreted by the anterior pituitary, it later became clear that it was a product of the placenta; it was named human chorionic gonadotropin, or HCG.

As the name implies, this hormone is produced by the chorion and has a gonadotropic effect. It is a glycoprotein substance with a molecular weight of *ca.* 30,000 and it can be detected in maternal blood and urine very early after fertilisation, about ten days after ovulation and five days before the expected time of onset of menstrual bleeding had fertilisation not taken place. In view of the fact that there is only the one source, the ovum must begin to produce HCG very soon after fertilisation and before implantation is complete.

The level of the hormone in the serum (and urine) rises in the first weeks of pregnancy to reach a peak during the third month and then falls sharply to a sixth of the peak value by four months. This level tends to remain fairly constant, with a secondary less marked rise during the last three months of pregnancy.

The role attributed to HCG is a luteotropic one. It is held to be the stimulus which prevents the regression of the corpus luteum when fertilisation has occurred, and also brings about the continued growth of the corpus luteum and the secretion of progesterone in the early weeks of pregnancy until the placental secretion obviates the need for such luteal activity. The administration of HCG has been shown to stimulate secretory activity of the corpus luteum (as assessed by the excretion of pregnanediol) and to increase the length of the luteal phase of the menstrual cycle, although it does not seem able to act on a corpus luteum that is already regressing. Many of the studies of the effects of HCG have necessarily been conducted on non-primates, but in monkeys prolongation of the life of the corpus luteum under its influence is accompanied by histological changes similar to those found in early pregnancy. The essential role of the corpus luteum in man and other primates however is limited to early pregnancy, and this poses the problem of what part HCG plays in the last six months of gestation.

Follicle stimulating effects of HCG have also been reported, particularly with high dosages, and the secretion of a second trophoblastic hormone has been suggested to explain this. In normal women the placental and pituitary hormones might act synergistically to produce more than one effect on the ovary. Even if HCG acts primarily on the ovary when present at a high level in plasma it is likely to influence not only the anterior pituitary, but other secretory tissues, both maternal and fetal. HCG might also exert an effect on the metabolism of steroids by the placenta, but although evidence for this has been published, it is difficult at present to fit such an action into any acceptable scheme. The secretion of HCG by the placenta however may well be influenced by fetal hormones, as the levels of HCG during later pregnancy tend to be significantly lower in women bearing male fetuses than in those bearing females.

Source of HCG

There is no doubt that HCG is produced by the trophoblast, but there is still some dispute as to whether the syncytiotrophoblast or the cytotrophoblast is the site of synthesis. Structurally the cytotrophoblast, as seen by light microscopy, bears more resemblance to other hormone-synthesising tissues than the syncytial elements; but electron microscopy shows that the latter contain an abundance of components, such as rough endoplasmic reticulum, commonly associated with the synthesis of secretory protein rather than with protein for cell multiplication. Histochemical studies aimed at identifying the carbohydrate moiety of HCG suggested that this might be localised in the cytotrophoblast of early but not late placentae, although positive reactions for carbohydrate (excluding glycogen) have been found in the syncytial layer. Probably observations of this kind are not valid as the amounts of hormone, and its carbohydrate fraction, are likely to be too small to be demonstrated histochemically. Immunocytochemical methods have indicated the syncytial tissue as the site of production. The close relationship between cytotrophoblast and syncytiotrophoblast, the latter developing from the former, perhaps suggests that synthetic activity might begin in the cytotrophoblastic stage and continue after its transformation to syncytium.

Growth-lactogenic-hormone

The presence of placental prolactin-like activity has been known since the mid 1930s, but convincing evidence for the occurrence of a substance or substances showing growth and lactogenic effects has mostly accumulated since the early 1960s. Probably the placenta secretes a single compound having both these properties.

A variety of names have been given to this factor: human chorionic growth hormone-prolactin (HCGP); human chorionic somatomammotropin (HCS); and human placental lactogen (HPL). The last of these terms is used in this text, bearing in mind the possibility that effects attributed to this single compound might yet prove to be due to two separate ones.

HPL has been conclusively shown to be synthesised by placental tissue. It is found in maternal blood and urine only during pregnancy, and disappears

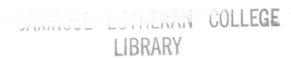

within a day of two of parturition. It has been extracted from trophoblast and from cultured placental tissue; immunofluorescent studies suggest that it originates in the syncytiotrophoblast. The purified substance has been reported to have a molecular weight of 19,000-30,000, although higher values have been proposed. It has been shown to have lactogenic properties, inducing lactation in rabbits and producing crop-sac activity in pigeons similar to that found following administration of LTH, and to exert lactogenic stimuli on cultured mouse mammary gland. Effects similar to growth hormone have been found in studies using the rat tibial test and uptake of radioactive sulphate by costal cartilage. In addition a luteotropic effect has been observed following administration of HPL to pseudo-pregnant hypophysectomised rats

The role of this compound in human pregnancy is far from clear. The plasma concentrations increase fairly closely in line with placental growth, and at term a secretion of up to 1.5g/24 h has been suggested. Most of the hormone is found in maternal blood and in the placenta, and very small amounts in fetal blood, amniotic fluid and maternal urine. Its lactogenic properties suggest that it may play a part, probably acting synergistically with other factors such as STH and LTH, in stimulating development of mammary tissue. Any luteotropic action would be expected to be limited to the early phase of pregnancy. Studies on animals indicate that it is not equivalent to STH, and although high doses promote nitrogen retention, there is some doubt as to whether HPL is responsible for the nitrogen retention which occurs in pregnancy. It may act on the placenta with HCG and play a part in the maintenance of placental secretion of oestrogen and progesterone, an activity in which, as already discussed, the placenta acts largely independently of extra-placental regulation.

The role of the placenta in producing other hormones is uncertain. Some secretion of ACTH has been proposed but not proven. The synthesis of MSH (see p. 3) has also been suggested and, although extracts of placenta have been shown to have MSH-like activity, the evidence for a placental secretion of this hormone is not strong. There are however some indications that a human chorionic thyrotropin (HCT) may be produced and secreted into the maternal circulation.

The morphology of the placenta varies greatly in different species. In the opossum, in which gestation lasts only 12-13 days, a yolk sac placenta develops. Hormonal control of gestation is largely by prolongation of the luteal phase of the oestrous cycle and the time of parturition corresponds to that of involution of the corpora lutea. In higher mammals the pattern of distribution of chorionic villi characterises the placenta of different species. These may be diffusely arranged as in the pig; form a girdle (zonary placenta) as in the bitch; be concentrated in one or more discs (discoid) as in monkeys; or lie in scattered rosettes (cotyledons) as in the cow. Placentae are also classified according to the degree of approximation of the maternal and fetal blood, from epithelio-chorial, in which there is simple apposition of the epithelial covering of the chorion and that lining the uterus, to haemo-endothelial in which the endothelium of the chorionic vessels is bathed in maternal blood.

Hormonal aspects of placentation also vary considerably in different species, and the variations in relative importance of the placenta and the corpora lutea have already been noted. In the pregnant mare a specific equine gonadotropin appears in the serum about the 40th day of pregnancy and increases in amount to about the 120th, then declines. This substance, PMS, is practically absent from the urine. It acts like a mixture of FSH and LH, and stimulates the development of large vesicular ovarian follicles, some of which ovulate and then undergo luteinisation while others form corpora lutea without ovulating. This gonadotropin is secreted by the uterine cups, structures of maternal origin.

Pregnancy Tests

The production of HCG by the placenta is used as a test for pregnancy, and such tests rely on the fact that plasma levels are high enough to give a positive test at about 10 days after the first missed period. A typical example is the 'Prepurex' (Wellcome) slide test: polystyrene latex particles sensitized with HCG will be agglutinated rapidly by antiserum to HCG. If urine from a pregnant woman (containing HCG) is mixed with the antiserum before the latex suspension is added, the antiserum will be neutralised and will be unable to agglutinate the latex particles; therefore **no agglutination** is a **positive** test, while the occurrence of **agglutination** indicates a **negative** test.

One does not expect a positive slide test until about two weeks after a missed period or less than 30 days after conception. Recently, circulating levels of a pregnancy-specific beta-glycoprotein have been found in early pregnancy, enabling a diagnosis of pregnancy to be made some 16 days after ovulation. This protein is produced by the placental trophoblast and appears in the maternal urine; it is also of value in the assessment of fetal well-being late in pregnancy.

In recent years the possibility of monitoring the fetus *in utero* has led to considerable obstetric and social advances. It is now, therefore, feasible for the obstetrician to assess the state of the fetus throughout pregnancy as well as to diagnose certain abnormalities. In the latter cases, termination of pregnancy may be advised where gross abnormality of the fetus is likely. Everyday examples would be a fetus affected by rubella virus, (or indeed exposed to rubella and therefore having a 30% chance of deformity), a fetus with severe spina bifida or with Down's syndrome. When we advance to the stage of being able to diagnose certain abnormalities which in themselves are not fatal but will result in deformity or mental deficiency, we enter an area of social obstetrics which will soon be a reality. The debate will centre on the choice offered to parents and whether appropriate action is taken. If only in a minority, some members of society will opt for the rights of the unborn child.

The following methods are currently used in assessing fetal mortality, fetal morbidity, intrauterine growth retardation and prematurity.

1. Clinical. Maternal factors such as age, parity, previous history and social class. Specific complications such as pre-eclampsia, rhesus incompatibility (now less of a problem with the advent of anti-D immunization), and medical complications such as heart disease and diabetes mellitus.
2. Electronic. The use of ultrasound.
3. Biochemical. Feto-placental hormones, enzymes, specific fetal proteins and phospholipids. Fetal/base status—using the estimation of the pH of fetal scalp blood.

The estimation of HPL, progesterone, oxytocinase and alpha-fetoprotein (the latter specifically for spina bifida) are the current interests of those concerned with fetal care.

Abortion. Various factors may lead to the premature loss of the conceptus from the uterus which occurs in abortion, including developmental anomalies of the maternal reproductive tract or of the embryo. In the light of what is known of the influence of hormones on the uterus, it seems clear that endocrine imbalance must also be considered important in this respect. Failure of the fertilised ovum to implant, for example, although not likely to be detected clinically, may follow insufficiency of the corpus luteum, as a result of which the decidua had failed to reach an appropriate progestational state for implantation.

Hormonal factors may also be associated with abortion in the post-implantation phase. The known role of progesterone in the maintenance of pregnancy suggested that an insufficiency of this hormone might lead to abortion and that, when abortion threatened, administration of progesterone might prevent its occurrence. An approach to the problem of women who suffer recurrent abortions has been to assess the level of progesterone secretion by determining the amounts of pregnanediol excreted—a procedure which requires repeated estimations to give any reliable assessment. There is evidence that abortion is more likely in women who show a low level of pregnanediol and hence a possibly inadequate trophoblastic function in the first trimester of pregnancy, but that it is not inevitable. Sequential measurements of the levels of HCG and HPL, if they show a failure to follow the normal incremental pattern in the early months, might also give some indication of the likelihood of loss of the conceptus.

Even if a deficiency in progesterone is a major factor in some abortions, the administration of progestogens will not necessarily reproduce the normal and prevent the outcome. Furthermore, some progestogens may produce virilisation of female fetuses, while attempts to prevent abortion by treatment with oestrogens carries the risk of the later development of vaginal cancers in female offspring.

Hydatidiform mole. This constitutes another disorder of pregnancy, relatively uncommon in Western countries (about 1 in 2500 pregnancies) but some ten times commoner in the East. In this condition the embryo either dies or fails to develop, but the tissue of the chorionic villi survives and proliferates, invading the uterine wall to a variable extent. The villi become distended with fluid, while the cells of the trophoblast continue to secrete HCG, resulting in high blood levels. Emboli of trophoblast commonly enter the bloodstream.

The histological structure of the invasive tissue and the extent of the invasion may vary greatly in different examples. A malignant condition resembling this in some respects is chorionic carcinoma, formerly carrying a high mortality but now often curable by chemotherapy.

PARTURITION

Factors influencing uterine contractility

Once pregnancy is established, the uterus usually remains quiescent for its duration. During the period of gestation the uterus increases greatly in volume as its contents grow, and there is a striking increase in the mass of uterine tissue, notably the muscle of its wall. At the end of gestation the uterus changes from a permissive organ, which had accommodated itself to the increasing size of its contents, to an actively contractile one which expels its contents in the process of birth, after which it rapidly involutes.

The duration of pregnancy, the period of gestation, varies over a wide range in different species, but it is remarkably constant within a single species. It lasts approximately 20 days in the common house mouse, 330 days in the horse and about 22 months in the African elephant. In women parturition usually occurs after about 267 days or 38 weeks. Despite many investigations it is still not clear what factors actually initiate parturition. In this as in other aspects of reproductive endocrinology, experimental studies on other mammals, and even on non-human primates, are not necessarily directly applicable to humans, since as already seen the endocrinology of pregnancy varies considerably between species.

Uterine muscle, the myometrium, is spontaneously contractile, even if it is completely denervated; furthermore it is potentially contractile throughout pregnancy, although its activity is normally prevented in some way until the fetuses have reached the appropriate stage of maturity to survive after birth. Quiescence during gestation might be due to a change in the properties of the myometrium itself, either an inhibition of the essential contractile mechanisms of the individual smooth muscle cells, or a block of the conduction of impulses from one cell to another, so that co-ordinated waves of contraction which are necessary for the expulsion of the uterine contents do not occur. Alternatively there might be some kind of barrier which prevents nervous stimuli reaching the uterus or a block to any hormones which might activate the myometrium. The latter effect could be brought about either by the prevention of the release of such hormones from their source or their inactivation before they could act on the myometrium.

Oestrogen and progesterone

From the earlier discussion of pregnancy it is clear that a change in progesterone and oestrogen secretion, or in the response of the uterus to the hormones, could be a factor in triggering off uterine contractions. In humans, the major site of production of the steroids shifts from the ovaries in early pregnancy to the placenta, which by virtue of its intimate association with the uterus is able to exert a local endocrine influence which is not necessarily reproducible by the systemic administration of progesterone or oestrogens. Fetal endocrine glands, notably the adrenals, are important for the production of C_{19} compounds utilised by the placenta in the production of oestrogens, so that increased fetal endocrine activity can influence placental synthesis of the latter hormones. Maternal adrenal corticoids must also be taken into account. The posterior pituitary hormone oxytocin, known to have the property of causing contraction of the smooth muscle of the reproductive tract, also needs to be assessed as a possible factor in the initiation of labour. Non-hormonal factors, notably the volume of the uterus, have been proposed as having an important influence on the timing of the onset of uterine contractions.

As already discussed, progesterone is essential for the establishment of pregnancy by conditioning the endometrium to a state in which implantation can occur and by suppressing the muscular contractions which would tend to expel any uterine contents. The importance of the latter effect is clearly shown by the abortion which follows ovariectomy (removal of the corpus luteum) in the critical phase of pregnancy in luteal dependent species. Progesterone seems to be essential for the maintenance of pregnancy in all species, although its source may be luteal, placental, or both of these. Hence a fall in the level of progesterone at the end of gestation might initiate labour by freeing the uterus from its inhibitory influence. In the rabbit for example ovariectomy during pregnancy is followed by uterine contractions sufficiently strong to crush and kill the fetuses; normally in this species the secretion of progesterone decreases in late pregnancy, although the gradual fall in level contrasts with the sudden onset of uterine contractions. This suggests that the reduction of progesterone is not in itself the trigger for the onset of parturition, but that a second factor, perhaps the release of oxytocin from the posterior pituitary, may be involved.

In other species, including man, the level of progesterone does not fall towards the end of the gestation period, but on the contary the highest levels are found at parturition. Figures for hormonal titres derived from blood samples or from urinary levels of progesterone metabolites do not however necessarily reflect the local concentrations of the hormone in the uterus, beneath and adjacent to the placenta.

Oestrogens, which as already noted are synthesised and secreted by the placenta, have several effects on the myometrium. Notably they increase its spontaneous rhythmic contractile activity and sensitivity to oxytocin, which progesterone inhibits. Hence it has been suggested that a rapid rise in oestrogen at the end of gestation could act as the trigger for parturition, oestrogen replacing progesterone as the dominant hormone influencing the uterus. Administration of oestrogens to pregnant women has not given a clear response, but some contractile effects have been noted.

The secretion of oestrogen increases as pregnancy advances and the highest level is reached just before parturition. In women, oestriol is the predominant substance. The ratio of urinary pregnanediol: oestriol increases from an early value of 100:1 to 3:1 at 20 weeks, and there is a gradual decrease in the later weeks of pregnancy. The increase in oestrogen secretion before parturition takes place gradually in primates, more rapidly in some other species. The fact that in women there is no acute change in the progesterone-oestrogen ratio suggests that a change in this ratio is not a main factor in the initiation of parturition.

Oxytocin

Oxytocin causes contractile activity of the myometrium when it is under the influence of oestrogen, and progesterone prevents this effect. During pregnancy the uterus does not contract in response to oxytocin, and the blood level of this hormone in women is low throughout pregnancy, rising appreciably only during the second stage of labour. ADH, which acts predominantly on the kidneys, but has a small oxytocic effect, is also released during labour. The sensitivity of the uterus to both oxytocin and ADH increases in later gestation, and most markedly at the end of gestation and during labour. In a study of the progesterone levels in the blood of women in whom oxytocin was used to induce labour, those who responded with regular uterine contractions within three hours had significantly lower levels of progesterone than those who did not so respond. In general the evidence seems to indicate that oxytocin is of importance only during labour, not in its initiation, and that increased sensitivity to the octapeptide due to progesterone withdrawal is not important to women.

Fetal factors

The role of the fetus and, as far as volume is concerned, of the fetal membranes and amniotic fluid, is another question which must be considered. Increased production of C_{19} adrenal cortical hormones is likely to be of significance in relation to rising levels of placental oestrogen, in view of the need for these to be supplied to the placenta before it can synthesise the latter hormone. Evidence that the fetal adrenals may play a significant part in the timing of parturition has been obtained for a number of mammalian species, but not for humans. In lambs, the fetal adrenals grow rapidly in the last week or so of pregnancy, and the blood levels of corticosteroids increase along with this growth. Fetal adrenalectomy or hypophysectomy (see p. 88) results in prolongation of pregnancy. In cattle, a deficiency of fetal 17-hydroxy-ketosteroids is associated with prolonged pregnancy and a flabby uterus which does not respond to oxytocin. Fetal adrenalectomy removes the source of glucocorticoids and of C_{19} oestrogen precursors, and since in these species cortisol probably does not cross the placenta, it is unlikely that fetal cortisol reaches the myometrium. Glucocorticoids may act as a specific stimulus for the initiation of parturition, and may also influence the production of steroids by the placenta.

As regards human pregnancies, evidence is necessarily indirect. Anencephalic fetuses in which the hypothalamus has not developed and the anterior pituitary is imperfect often have small adrenal glands with an underdeveloped cortex. Delayed onset of parturition has been correlated with the extent of the adrenal cortical deficiency. In cases of congenital adrenal hypoplasia there does not seem to be any clear trend towards prolongation of pregnancy, and the same appears to hold for congenital adrenal hyperplasia (see p. 90). In humans, cortisol can cross the placenta and increased secretion by the fetal adrenal of cortisol and C_{19} oestrogen precursors would result in increased placental synthesis of oestrogens. The administration of corticosteroids to pregnant women is followed by a fall in the amount of oestriol excreted in the urine, presumably following a fall in fetal ACTH and consequent depression of fetal adrenal cortical activity.

Uterine volume

Uterine volume may influence the initiation of parturition. Growth of the uterus seems to depend on the combined effects of the growth of the uterine contents producing distension and the simultaneous effects of progesterone and oestrogen on the myometrium. Under these influences the uterus grows throughout pregnancy with no increase in its resting tension, so that the contents are not subjected to undue mechanical stresses. Increase in volume may however be associated with increased excitability; hypertrophy certainly occurs. In non-humans, litter size in a given species may vary considerably more than the variation in time of gestation, and in women the size of the conceptus and hence of the uterus may vary widely with little variation in length of gestation; in twin pregnancies for example parturition occurs on average at 37 weeks, some five weeks after the weight of the fetuses equals that of a single conceptus. The uterus may be greatly enlarged by the occurrence of hydramnios, a condition in which the amount of amniotic fluid, which normally averages about 600 ml at term, is considerably increased to 2 litres or more. Distension of the uterus to this extent however advances the onset of labour by only about one week.

Relaxin

In many mammals relaxation of pelvic ligaments and laxity of the pelvic joints, notably the symphysis pubis, develops in late pregnancy and allows enlargement of the birth canal and eases the birth process. The effect is brought about by a hormone, relaxin. Probably a polypeptide, it occurs in the placenta, ovaries and blood during pregnancy, increasing in amount towards term. Its effects are more marked in some species than others, and it acts in conjunction with other hormones, notably oestrogen. It can be assayed by determining the degree of relaxation of the pubic symphysis, either by palpation or radiologically, in oestrogen-primed guinea pigs.

Relaxin is found in pregnancy blood even in species in which pelvic relaxation is not pronounced, but disappears after parturition. It also acts as an inhibitor of spontaneous uterine contractions in rodents, and in women has been found to inhibit uterine contractions in cases of premature labour. In combination with oestrogen it softens the cervix, and in rats and mice it has been found to act synergistically with oestrogen and progesterone in promoting growth of the virgin mammary glands.

In women, the onset of parturition occurs at a time when the maternal progesterone has reached a plateau, maternal oestrogen has gradually achieved a peak level and the fetal adrenal is actively secretory, producing corticoids and oestrogen precursors. Uterine volume appears to play no major part, and oxytocin is probably of little importance until labour is in progress. Several factors are involved and the whole mechanism underlying the initiation of labour is still unclear.

MAMMARY GLANDS AND LACTATION

Considerable increase in size of the breasts commonly takes place during adolescence, but before the first pregnancy the mammary tissue shows little evidence of its enormous secretory potential. At this time the breasts consist largely of fatty and fibrous tissue, although a rudimentary duct system is present. This consists of fifteen to twenty main ducts, each associated with a lobe of mammary tissue, which it will drain during lactation. The lobulation of the breast is emphasised by septa of connective tissue which extend deeply from the skin and delimit the territory of each main duct. Each of these ducts is dilated near its opening at the nipple to form a lactiferous sinus. The main ducts receive smaller secondary ducts, each of which will drain a lobule of secretory tissue. At this stage the only indication of secretory elements is in the form of scattered groups of cells associated with the secondary ducts, surrounded by abundant connective tissue which contains smooth muscle, some of which is arranged parallel to the main ducts.

Changes in pregnancy

The transformation of the inactive breast into an actively secretory one begins early in pregnancy and continues throughout gestation. The changes which occur are the development of secretory acini, extension and enlargement of the duct system to carry the secreted milk to the nipple, and a great increase in vascularity. From about the fifth week onwards, the breasts begin to enlarge and the increasing blood flow results in dilatation of superficial veins, which become more easily visible. The nipples increase in size, their areolae extend and particularly in the first pregnancy become darker due to increased pigmentation of the skin. At the same time small cutaneous glands, the glands of Montgomery which open on the areola, become more prominent and appear as small tubercles.

The microscopic changes begin early in pregnancy. During the first three months or so the epithelial cells of the smaller ducts begin to divide and new ducts extend into the surrounding connective tissue. These new formations become grouped together and the lobular pattern within the main lobes of the breast becomes more apparent. The secretory tissue develops mostly during the middle months of pregnancy by the outgrowth of buds of cells from the small ducts, which become canalised to form acini lined by a single layer of cuboidal epithelial cells.

The great increase in secretory components of the breast is accompanied by modifications in the connective tissue. The main septa become thinner, and the stroma which previously made up the bulk of the breast becomes modified into fairly thin investments for the closely packed acini. The connective tissue which originally invested the small ducts develops a rich network of capillary vessels, so that the developing acini, extending into this, gain a close relationship with the rich vascular supply necessary for the secretory process.

During the last third of pregnancy formation of new elements is less marked; the breasts still enlarge although less rapidly than before. Although secretory activity in the acini has usually begun earlier, it increases considerably during this phase. Both acini and ducts become distended with colostrum, a fluid precursor of milk which differs from it in having a higher content of globulin, non-fatty acids and chloride, and less lactose. Colostrum also carries immune bodies. It continues to be secreted, in larger amounts, in the immediate post-partum days until it is replaced by milk. Although development of the ducts and acini and the onset of secretory activity largely occur in different phases of pregnancy, there is some overlap, and also a wave of cellular proliferation occurs at the end of parturition or the onset of lactation.

As already noted, the breast contains some smooth muscle, but this is not the only contractile element present. As ducts and secretory acini grow another type of cell differentiates in the junctional zone between the epithelial cells and their investment of connective tissue. This is the myoepithelial cell, so called because it is both contractile and shows some epithelial features. Each of these cells consists of a body from which extend processes which embrace the acini and ducts, so that an incomplete layer of contractile elements lies beneath the secretory epithelium. Contraction of these myoepithelial cells (which, as described later, is under hormonal control) will assist in the expulsion of secretion from the acini and along ducts towards the nipple.

Lactation

The structure of the breast during lactation does not differ greatly from that during the last weeks of pregnancy. As already noted, colostrum is formed before birth of the child, and it continues to be secreted for a day or two after birth until it gives way to the secretion of milk.

During lactation, the mammary tissue retains the overall structure attained at the end of pregnancy, although the epithelial cells are taller and more basophilic. Electron microscopy shows an increase in the number of microvilli on the surface of the cells, increased amounts of rough endoplasmic reticulum and enlargement of the Golgi complex. Fat globules, which are already present in the secretory cells before parturition, are more numerous when lactation is established. Activity is not necessarily uniform throughout the whole breast at any one time; some areas are more actively secretory than others, and groups of acini may go through phases of high and low secretory activity.

At the end of lactation the breast begins to return to a resting condition. The secretory acini collapse and atrophy; the ducts become narrower and fibrous connective tissue and fat increase in amount as secretory elements disappear. There is no longer a need for a rich blood supply, and this decreases. Eventually the gland returns to a quiescent state with a microscopic appearance of a non-secretory tissue, although once lactation had occurred ducts and epithelial remnants remain a more prominent feature than before the first pregnancy; the nipples and areolae tend to be wider and darker; and the breasts often remain larger than they were before.

Hormones and mammary glands

The phases of growth and activity of the mammary glands described above are all dependent on hormonal stimuli which differ for each phase. The phases can be broadly designated as duct growth, lobulo-alveolar development, the onset of secretory activity and full lactation. The latter process has been subdivided (see Folley, 1940) as below

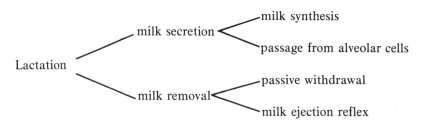

Milk contains sugar (lactose), fat and protein (casein, alpha- and beta-lactalbumin) and electrolytes (sodium, potassium, calcium, chloride and bicarbonate). It is therefore scarcely surprising that a number of hormones with general metabolic effects, such as insulin and adrenal corticoids, as well as some with particular associations with the reproductive system, influence lactation.

As with so many other aspects of hormones and reproduction, the basic understanding of the factors involved in mammary growth and secretion have been largely obtained from experimental work on animals and applied to women, where possible taking account of hormonal changes throughout pregnancy, pathological states and the observed effects of the administration of various hormonal compounds. Species differences are considerable; but regardless of its source, mammary tissue is influenced by oestrogen and progesterone, by adrenal and placental steroids, and by thyroxine and insulin. Necessarily, the pituitary tropic hormones controlling the appropriate target organs are therefore involved—FSH, LH, ACTH and TSH. The metabolic hormone STH also exerts an effect, and a major pituitary influence is exercised by means of LTH (prolactin). The placenta, as well as its contribution of steroids, also secretes the lactogenic hormone HPL, also referred to as human chorionic growth hormone-prolactin (HCGP), briefly considered on p. 58.

Oestrogen, in the presence of STH and adrenal steroids, stimulates growth of the mammary duct system. In some animals this seems to be the limit of its effect, and the addition of progesterone is necessary for the development of lobulo-alveolar growth. In other species, however, possibly including primates, oestrogen alone can produce both duct and lobulo-alveolar growth. The presence of insulin is important for the process of epithelial proliferation and development of the lobulo-alveolar pattern.

The effect of oestrogen on mammary tissue is demonstrated by the growth of the main duct system which occurs at puberty and also, in the absence of pregnancy, in the proliferative and regressive changes which occur with the phases of the menstrual cycle. When pregnancy occurs, the increasing levels of oestrogen and progesterone stimulate the progressive development of both the duct system and the acinar secretory tissue.

LTH (prolactin) and placental lactogen

Pituitary lactotropic hormone (prolactin) in women exercises a major effect on the initiation and maintenance of lactation. A hormone with close affinities to LTH occurs in a wide range of species including birds, fishes and reptiles. Although this cannot exert any lactotropic activity in non-mammals, it gives positive results with the traditional bioassay methods for LTH, such as growth of the pigeon crop sac and growth of rabbit mammary tissue after injection of the hormone into a duct. In migratory fish such as salmon which leave the sea to spawn in the fresh inland waters, prolactin induces sodium retention by the gills when the fish return to fresh water; in birds it induces broodiness and nest building, and in mammals maternal behaviour. In a few species it has been shown to have a luteotropic action, prolonging the life of the corpus luteum, a property which led to the use of the term luteotropin for LTH, which although justifiable for the rat is not widely applicable. The hormone also occurs in males.

The separate existence of LTH in humans has been conclusively shown only relatively recently. Previously it was generally considered that it was identical with STH, and that the same molecule had both growth and lactogenic effects. The development of sensitive and specific methods of assay, notably radioimmunoassay, contributed importantly to the recognition that two distinct hormones exist. A similar confusion applied to the cellular origin of the hormone in the anterior pituitary. In view of the fact that the pituitary glands of non-pregnant women contain only about one fifteenth as much LTH as STH, this is perhaps not surprising. During pregnancy and lactation the amount of LTH increases considerably, and this is correlated with the appearance of a large number of "pregnancy" cells in the gland. The application of immunofluorescence techniques has shown that LTH is localised in these cells.

LTH is a polypeptide hormone distinct not only from STH, but also chemically from HPL. During pregnancy the level of LTH begins to rise about the eighth week and continues to rise until delivery. If suckling does not follow, the level falls to pre-pregnancy values within a few weeks. If the child is suckled, a raised level of about twice that in non-pregnant women is maintained, and once breast feeding is established this level rises tenfold or more in response to suckling. After some months, the level falls to non-pregnant levels, and suckling does not elicit a rise.

Placental lactogen in women also increases in amount throughout pregnancy from about the sixth week onwards. This increase parallels that of LTH, although the amount of HPL/ml may be thirty-fold or so greater than that of LTH at term.

It has been shown for several species that both LTH and HPL act synergistically with other hormones on the developing mammary tissue during pregnancy, and make at any rate some contribution to the development of the lobulo-alveolar system. The main action of both of these hormones however seems to be the stimulation of the secretion of milk, namely their lactogenic effect. Yet despite the high levels of each towards the end of pregnancy, lactation does not occur until after parturition. One explanation of this is that the high titres of oestrogen and progesterone during later pregnancy block the action of the lactogens on mammary tissue and thus prevent secretion of milk. The rapid fall in both oestrogens and progesterone after parturition allows the lactogens to act, and secretion of milk follows the initial production of colostrum. Another hypothesis invokes the lactogenic effect of oestrogen, which stimulates the secretion of LTH by the anterior pituitary, an effect which may be inhibited by progesterone. After parturition the absolute fall in level of both types of steroid accompanied by a fall in progesterone relative to oestrogen perhaps allows the lactogenic effect of the latter to assert itself. This takes no account of the action of HPL. The administration of large doses of oestrogen to women in the post-partum period can effectively block lactation without reducing the levels of LTH, which supports the theory that oestrogen acts directly on the mammary tissue.

The maintenance of lactation depends on suckling, and if milk is not removed from the breast, lactation ceases. It also ceases if the pituitary gland of lactating animals is removed and can then be restored by giving pituitary hormones, notably LTH and STH. Lack of adrenal cortical hormones results in a diminished secretion of milk, and although in some species (e.g. cow) the administration of corticoids to intact animals suppresses lactation, the adrenal cortex generally seems to contribute to the hormonal background necessary for normal lactation. The presence of the thyroid gland is not essential, although without it the amount of secretion and its duration are reduced. Studies in women, as well as in animals, have however shown that the administration of TSH is followed by a marked increase in serum LTH which in women is followed by engorgement of the breasts.

Milk ejection reflex, hypothalamus and pituitary

An important aspect of suckling is the active ejection of the milk lying in the deeper parts of the duct system and alveoli and not readily available to the sucking child. The flow of milk into the child's mouth indeed depends not on the amount of suction applied to the breast, but on the back pressure within the secretory acini and ducts. The chief part played by the child is to empty the teat which is formed from the mother's breast by sucking the nipple to the back of the mouth, occluding its base and stripping its contents by applied positive pressure; suction is of only secondary importance, and milk may continue to flow from the nipple if the child is removed from the breast.

The myoepithelial cells which lie around the alveoli and ducts have already been described. These cells contract under the influence of the posterior pituitary hormone, oxytocin, which is released from the infundibular process into the blood as a reflex response to the stimulus of putting the child to the breast. The hormone passes to the mammary tissue and there exerts its action on the contractile cells, so that milk is expelled from the alveoli and along the ducts towards the nipple. The effect may be so marked that milk spurts from the nipple even before the child has begun to suck. The removal of the neurohypophysis, or transection of the nerve fibres of the pituitary stalk, will prevent this reflex release of oxytocin. In addition to the contraction of myoepithelial cells, smooth muscle within the breast also contracts and plays a part in milk ejection.

The anterior pituitary is of course concerned with a number of target organs or tissues, and the hypothalamus is involved in the control of the secretion of the appropriate tropic hormones. The release of LTH in greater amounts during pregnancy and lactation involves an inhibition of the normal secretion of the "prolactin inhibiting factor", PIF, into the portal blood since, although inhibiting factors have been isolated for some of the other anterior pituitary hormones, LTH seems to be the only one in which inhibition is the predominant method for control of its secretion. This is emphasised by the finding that in pituitary glands transplanted away from the median eminence, the hormones of the pars distalis are all secreted in greatly reduced amounts with the exception of LTH, whose output increases. The cytology of such transplants is in keeping with this and the LTH cells are the only ones to retain their normal characteristics in ectopic sites.

The LTH released during suckling may inhibit the typical sequential pattern of release of FSH and LH on which normal menstrual cycles depend. Amenorrhoea commonly follows parturition: it may last a relatively short time, two months or so, but if a child continues to be suckled it may extend for much longer periods of about a year; if menstrual cycles do appear during long-continued lactation, they tend to be irregular. The rate of pregnancy (if contraception is not practised) is low, of the order of 10% in women lactating for 9 months or more, compared with 75% in women not breast feeding. During the post-partum period, women do not respond to the administration of LH/FSH-RH with the anticipated rise in the output of FSH and LH, and this effect lasts longer in women who continue to lactate. This observation indicates a direct inhibitory effect on the pituitary but does not rule out a similar effect on the hypothalamus. The intermittent surges of LTH released during suckling may thus interfere with the hypothalamic secretion of LH/FSH-RH, or directly inhibit the secretion of FSH and LH by the anterior pituitary. A further factor in the "contraceptive" effect of lactation and suckling may be an insensitivity of the ovary to the gonadotropic hormones, so that cyclical changes are either suppressed or, if they occur, ovulation is lacking.

Lactotropic hormones may act on the fetus and newborn child. The secretion of "witches milk" from the nipples of newborn children is commonly referred to as indicative of hormonal stimulation of mammary tissue in the fetus during late fetal life. A high level of LTH, coupled with the fall in oestrogen in the fetal blood after birth, could account for this transitory false lactation from secretory tissue which soon regresses and remain inactive until the time of puberty.

LTH occurs in large amounts in the amniotic fluid and is probably derived from the placenta. In the first trimester its concentration is several hundred fold greater than in maternal or fetal plasma, but as plasma levels rise this ratio falls, reaching a value of 3 or 4:1 at term. Although the significance of the presence of the hormone in amniotic fluid is not clear, it has been suggested that it might exert a somatotropic effect or perphaps act, as in migratory fish, to modify the ionic content of the fluid.

6

Fetal Endocrine Activity

During intrauterine life fetal endocrine glands develop and begin to secrete. As already seen, the fetal adrenal cortex is an important source of hormones utilised by the placenta in the synthesis of steroids. Fetal hormones also play a role in fetal metabolism and growth, and the gonadal hormones, notably in genetically male fetuses, are of great importance for the normal development of the reproductive system and, by acting on central nervous structures, for the development of typical behavioural patterns.

Present knowledge of the functional importance of fetal endocrine glands has been derived from studies of the histology, ultrastructure and histochemistry of fetal endocrines and from assays of hormones in tissues and blood. The classical technique of ablation of an endocrine organ, to study the results of a deficiency of its secretions, understandably proved difficult to apply to small mammals *in utero*, but Alfred Jost and his colleagues introduced a technique for fetal hypophysectomy of rats and rabbits. The procedure was the apparently crude one of decapitation *in utero*, but the use of appropriate controls indicated its validity and showed that the technique could provide valuable information on prenatal pituitary activity. More refined techniques have permitted the destruction of the pituitary gland *in situ* and, particularly in large animals, such as sheep, operative removal of the adrenals and thyroid has been carried out, the fetuses then being allowed to remain *in utero*. Removal of the gonads and implants of these organs have played a major part in the understanding of the factors underlying development of the reproductive tract. As regards man, observations of fetal malformations involving endocrine organs have enabled some correlations with the results of experimental studies, and the amounts of hormones in blood and tissue have been assayed.

The fetal pituitary is active from an early stage in gestation. In humans secretion begins during the second month, and during intrauterine life the anterior part of the gland secretes STH, LH, TSH, ACTH and LTH, while ADH and oxytocin are synthesised and secreted by the hypothalamo-neuro-hypophysial system. Fetal hypophysectomy of experimental animals has shown particularly clearly that pituitary hormones act on specific target organs and take part in the control of activity of the developing gonads, thyroid and adrenal cortices.

Jost has suggested that the development of a given endocrine gland can be considered in three stages. The first is that of morphological differentiation;

the second, the acquisition by the tissue of the biochemical capacity for the production of hormones; the third, the actual synthesis and release of hormones, that is the achievement of complete secretory activity. In those endocrine glands normally under the control of pituitary tropic hormones it seems likely that the third stage is dependent on the appropriate tropic hormone being present.

As far as the adenohypophysis is concerned the assumption of fully integrated activity involves the development of hypothalamic control. This requires not only the maturation of those neural elements concerned with the elaboration and secretion of hypothalamic releasing hormones, but also the formation of the portal vascular link which delivers these factors to the gland. In rats and rabbits the portal system does not develop until late in gestation, and the primary and secondary capillary beds are not fully formed until early postnatal life; but release of tropic hormones from the adenohypophysis seems to occur before this process is complete.

GONADS AND REPRODUCTIVE ORGANS

Development

Sex is genetically determined and established at the time of fertilisation. The female germ cells all have the same haploid complement of chromosomes, in humans 22 autosomes and one sex chromosome, X. The spermatozoa are of two kinds, each with 22 autosomes, but one carrying an X chromosome, the other a Y. Since an XX complement is characteristic of females, fertilisation of an ovum by an X-carrying spermatozoon will result in the development of a femal embryo with a diploid chromosomal complement of 46, XX. A Y chromosome however dictates the development of a male embryo, regardless of the presence of a single X component, and fertilisation of an ovum by a 22, Y-carrying spermatozoon will result in a 46, XY, male embryo. Abnormal complements of chromosomes are associated with abnormal development, and certain endocrine syndromes with a chromosomal basis are considered on p. 92.

The normal development of internal and external organs of reproduction depends in part on chromosomal sex and in part on the presence or absence of hormones of the fetal testis. In order to appreciate the relative importance of these factors and some of the possible results of maldevelopment, the essential embryology of male and femal reproductive systems is briefly considered.

Internal reproductive organs

The reproductive system consists of three essential elements; the testes or ovaries producing the germ cells; the ducts which transport the germ cells and, in the female, provide for the development of the embryo; and the external organs of reproduction.

The gonads, the initially undifferentiated sex glands which will produce both germ cells and hormones first appear in human embryos of about 6 mm CR length during the fifth week of development, as ventro-medial thickenings of the two urogenital ridges. The latter are masses of tissue which lie on either side of the midline on the dorsal abdominal wall and, as the name implies, are associated with the development of the urinary system as well as reproductive structures (Fig. 13). Each thickened region soon forms a

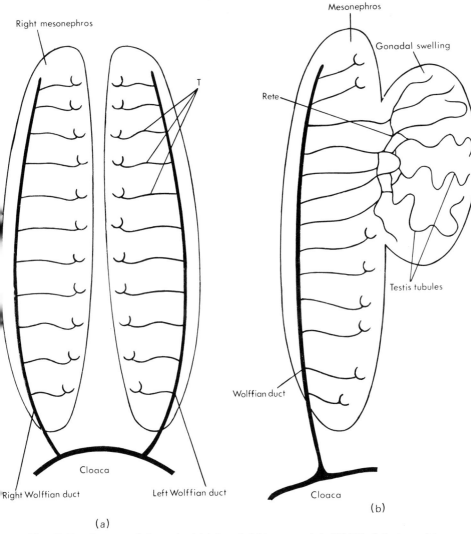

Fig. 13. Development of the testis. (a) left and right mesonephric (Wolffian) ducts receiving mesonephric tubules (T) and draining to the cloaca; (b) development of gonadal tissue shown in relation to one mesonephros. Primitive testis tubules connect via a primitive rete with some of the mesonephric tubules and thence with the Wolffian duct.

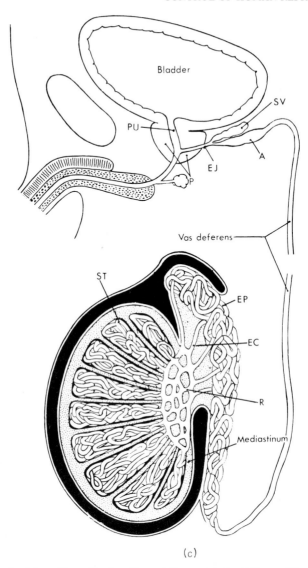

(c)

Fig. 13c. The final disposition of testis with seminiferous tubules (ST) rete (R) and efferent canaliculi (EC) draining into the duct of the epididymis (EP), which is continuous with the vas deferens. (A-ampulla of vas; EJ-ejaculatory duct; P-prostate; PU-prostatic urethra,) SV-seminal vesicle.

secondary ridge bulging medially into the coelom, at which stage it constitutes the genital ridge. This soon becomes shorter, and the original broad attachment to the urinary part of the dorsal ridge of tissue (the mesonephric ridge) forms a much thinner mesentery.

The mesonephric ridge on each side gives rise to the mesonephros, a transient primitive kidney which serves as a temporary excretory organ to a variable extent in different species.

In genetically male embryos the gonadal swellings begin to differentiate into testes at about the 15 mm stage, when the embryo is in its seventh week. In genetically female embryos distinctive ovarian features do not become evident until several weeks later than males, so that the "indifferent" stage is prolonged. Testicular differentiation is marked by the formation of cords of cells, the testis cords, in the central region of the gonad and the development of a layer of tissue enclosing these which becomes the fibrous capsule, or tunica albuginea. This is covered externally at first by a "germinal" epithelium. The testis cords become arranged so that they converge towards the attachment of the mesentery (the mesorchium), where the rete, part of the duct system carrying spermatozoa from the testis, is developing. The cords of cells are the forerunners of the seminiferous tubules, which do not develop fully into tubules until puberty. Between the cords of cells connective tissue forms the framework of the testis, carrying blood vessels and lymphatics. Clumps of specialised cells develop in this connective tissue to form the testicular interstitial or Leydig cells, which are secretory in both fetal and postnatal life.

The duct system of the testis in mammals is essentially developed by the taking over of some of the tubules and the duct of the primitive mesonephric kidney (Fig. 13). The mesonephros on each side consists of a series of tubules, more or less S-shaped in transverse sections. The medial part of each tubule is closely associated with a leash of thin-walled blood vessels with which it forms a primitive filtration unit. Laterally, each tubule opens into a duct which runs longitudinally in a cephalo-caudal direction to open into the urogenital sinus. This is the mesonephric or Wolffian duct. Each definitive or permanent kidney in mammals is formed from a later developing meta-nephros into which grows the ureteric bud, an outgrowth of the terminal lower part of the mesonephric duct.

A connection occurs between some of the cranial mesonephric tubules and the ducts of the rete testis about the sixth month of intrauterine life. These mesonephric tubules then become the efferent ductules of the epididymis, and establish a link between the future seminiferous tubules and rete tubules of the testis, and the Wolffian duct. The cranial part of the latter becomes the convoluted duct of the epididymis and the caudal part the ductus (vas) deferens, which ends as the ejaculatory duct opening into the prostatic urethra. The seminal vesicle develops as an outgrowth from the terminal part of the mesonephric duct. In female embryos the mesonephric ducts largely disappear.

The oviducts arise from secondary structures which develop for this specific purpose. These are the Müllerian or paramesonephric ducts, each of which forms as a groove in the mesonephric mass lateral to the mesonephric duct, first appearing in both male and female embryos at about the 10 mm stage, or six weeks. Each duct originates cranially and progresses caudally; its cranial end remains open but the rest closes to form the duct. In male embryos only small remnants of the Müllerian system persist.

Caudally, near the cloaca, the left and right urogenital ridges fuse to form the genital cord, and the elongating Müllerian ducts come to lie together within this mass of tissue, having crossed in front of the mesonephric duct of each side. The Müllerian ducts thus persist as distinct right and left-sided structures in their upper part, but fuse caudally (Fig. 14). The fused portions form the uterus, cervix and part of the vagina.

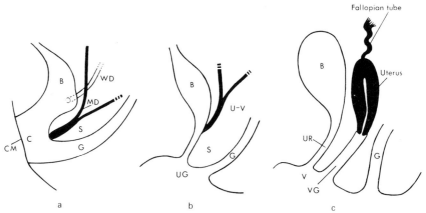

Fig. 14. Summary of the development of the internal female reproductive organs; the definitive ureter is not shown (a) the cloaca (C) closed by the cloacal membrane (CM) communicates with the future bladder (B) which receives the Wolffian duct (WD), and with the terminal gut (G). The lower ends of the Müllerian ducts (MD) have fused and lie in the incomplete septum (S) between the urinary and alimentary organs; (b) the cloacal membrane has now broken down and the septum separates urogenital and alimentary parts of the former cloaca. There is a urogenital sinus (UG) into which the bladder and the utero-vagina (U-V) open; (c) further development gives separate openings of the urethra (UR) and vagina (VG) into the vestibule (V).

External genitalia

The external genitalia as well as the internal organs pass through an indifferent stage and since hormones play an important part in the later differentiation of typically male or female features, the embryological changes are briefly considered here.

Non-placental vertebrates have a cloaca, a common chamber which receives both the faecal material from the gut and the genito-urinary products. In placental vertebrates this common chamber becomes divided into an anterior urogenital and a posterior faecal part, although the embryos pass through a cloacal stage. Male placental vertebrates develop a penis, which serves for the introduction of sperm into the female genital tract as well as for the passage of urine.

The critical phase as far as hormonal influences are concerned begins with the cloacal stage of embryological development. The cloaca is transformed by the growth of a transverse urorectal or cloacal septum into an anterior and posterior division (Fig. 14); in the human embryo this is completed by the seventh week. The anterior division forms the bladder superiorly and the urogenital sinus inferiorly. By complex changes, the ureters (which originated as outgrowths from the lower parts of the mesonephric ducts) come to open into the upper (vesical) part of the cavity, and the mesonephric and fused Müllerian ducts into the lower urogenital part; the latter consists of a pelvic part continuous via a narrow short segment with the bladder and a phallic part distal to this. In the female, the short connecting segment forms the permanent urethra, while the pelvic and phallic parts of the urogenital sinus form the vestibule, into which both the urinary and genital tracts open (Fig. 14). In the male, the homologue of the female urethra is the upper part of the prostatic urethra, extending from the bladder to the seminal colliculus, a swelling in the posterior wall where the two ejaculatory ducts open. The pelvic part of the urogenital sinus forms the lower part of the prostatic urethra and the membranous urethra; the phallic part of the sinus forms the spongy, penile urethra.

A remnant of the Müllerian system persists in males as a small midline diverticulum opening onto the seminal colliculus. This is the utriculus masculinus or prostatic utricle. Although in monkeys it has been shown to undergo histological changes in response to hormonal influence, it does not appear to have any functional significance in man.

The prostate gland in the male develops as numerous outgrowths of urethral epithelium into the connective tissue surrounding the urethra, and the bulbo-urethral glands also grow out as epithelial buds from the future first part of the cavernous urethra. In the female the vestibular glands of Bartholin, which are the equivalent of the male bulbo-urethral glands, arise from the equivalent part of the urogenital sinus.

During the fifth to seventh week of human embryonic development the external genitalia have a sexually indifferent form (Fig. 15). At first there is an anterior midline genital tubercle, and caudal to this a shallow groove flanked on either side by slightly raised urogenital folds and floored by the thin urogenital membrane. At the posterior (anal) extremity of the groove is the area in which the urorectal septum has joined the cloacal membrane. Later, but still in an indifferent stage, the genital tubercle enlarges to form a rudimentary phallus and rounded genital swellings develop on each side. The urogenital membrane ruptures, so that the urogenital sinus opens externally at the base of the phallus (Fig. 16).

Essentially, the general form of female external genitalia is now complete. The shallow cavity which has opened to the anterior by the breakdown of the urogenital membrane forms the vestibule; the two flanking urogenital folds which lie on each side of the slit-like opening form the labia minora, and the

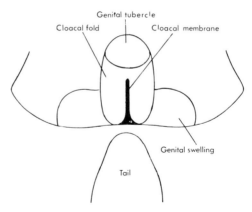

Fig. 15. The external genitalia at the early indifferent stage of development. Cloacal folds surround the cloacal membrane. Anteriorly the folds continue into a genital tubercle, and laterally lie the genital swellings.

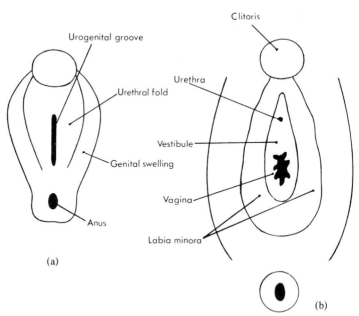

Fig. 16. The later stages of development of the female external genitalia. (a) by about mid-term a midline urogenital groove is flanked by urethral folds and more laterally by the genital swellings. A separate anus is now present; (b) at birth, the urethra and vagina now open into the vestibule, which is bounded by the labia minora. Laterally the labia majora have developed from the genital swellings and the genital tubercle has become transformed into the clitoris.

more lateral genital swellings, the labia majora. Anteriorly the genital tubercle develops into the clitoris, and the opening of the vestibule is limited posteriorly by the primary perineum where the urorectal septum fused with the cloacal membrane. The urethra and the vagina both open separately into the vestibule. This definitive stage is established by ten weeks, and although considerable changes in relative size and position of internal and external genitalia continue after this, the essential anatomical relationships of the mature female are established by this time.

The formation of the male external genitalia is basically a process of differentiation from the indifferent and essentially female condition (Fig. 17). Briefly, the development consists of a progressive fusion of the edges of the urogenital groove extending forwards to the genital tubercle, so that the urogenital sinus is transformed into an elongated urethral tube, destined to become the spongy urethra. Meanwhile the genital swellings move relatively posteriorly and become transformed into the two scrotal swellings, each of which will form one half of the scrotum, their line of fusion remaining marked as the scrotal raphé. The genital tubercle forms, proximally, the

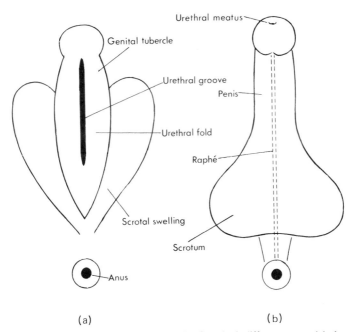

(a)   (b)

Fig. 17. Development of the male external genitalia after the indifferent stage. (a) the genital tubercle is developing into the phallus. In the midline is the urethral groove, bordered by the urethral folds. The lateral genital swellings are now scrotal swellings; (b) by the time of birth the penis is fully formed, and the urethral groove has closed to give the penile urethra which opens at the meatus. The line of fusion shows a midline raphé. The scrotal swellings have also fused to form the scrotum.

shaft of the penis, while its distal part enlarges and forms the glans. Finally, the urethral groove closes along the whole length of the shaft, and by a combination of grooving and canalisation the urethra finally extends to open at the tip of the glans.

Gradually during intrauterine life the ovaries or testes descend from their original position. In the female, the ovaries and their associated tubes come to lie within the pelvis; in the male the testes normally enter the scrotum before birth.

HORMONES AND SEXUAL DIFFERENTIATION

Certain hormones influence some aspects of the normal developmental process outlined above, and abnormalities of the hormonal environment at certain critical stages can result in permanent anatomical and functional derangements of the reproductive system. Hormonal influences exerted at a non-critical phase may produce changes in organs which persist only as long as the stimulus is exerted.

As already noted, genetic sex is established at fertilisation. An XY embryo develops a gonadal primordium which at first (at about 6 mm CR length) is not histologically recognisable as testis or ovary, but which becomes recognisable as a testis about three weeks later, at the seventh or eighth week, 15-17 mm stage, before sexual differentiation of the genital tract can be recognised. Differentiation of recognisable ovaries in genetically female (XX) embryos does not occur until a considerably later stage of embryonic development. Testicular differentiation depends on influence exerted by the Y chromosome on the indifferent gonad, directing it by some means as yet unknown. In the absence of such direction the indifferent gonad develops into an ovary.

While the factors influencing the development of a testis are not entirely clear, others which play a major role in the differentiation of the genital ducts have been well established, of necessity largely by observations on animals. In one strain of rabbits differentiation of the genital tract occurs progressively from the 20th day after insemination. If male fetuses are castrated *in utero* before day 19, no male characteristics develop. The mesonephric ducts disappear while the Müllerian ducts remain and develop into oviducts, uterus and that part of the vagina which is usually formed from them in female fetuses. In such castrates the external genitalia also fail to develop into the male form.

Not all parts of the developing male genital tract are sensitive to the lack of testicular hormones at the same time, but different components pass through different critical periods. Castration before a critical stage for a given component is reached prevents its development along the typical male line, while castration after this critical stage does not interfere with masculine differentiation. In the rabbits referred to above, castration of fetuses before day 22 is necessary to prevent development of the two anterior prostatic buds, and before day 23 to prevent that of the rest of the prostate, seminal vesicles and male external genitalia. The vas deferens fails to develop after castration just before day 24, but if the operation is delayed to day 24 or later all features of the male reproductive tract appear, although they may be smaller than normal.

By comparison with male fetuses, removal of the ovaries at any stage does not prevent the development of any of the features of the female genital tract. The possibility that maternal hormones crossing the placenta compensate for the fetal ovaries has been ruled out by the demonstration that *in vitro* preparations of fetal tissue showed persistence of Müllerian ducts and disappearance of Wolffian ducts, even when pieces of genetically male reproductive tract were used.

Thus, although sexual differentiation of the gonads into testes or ovaries seems to be primarily dependent on chromosomal make-up, the later differentiation of the genital tract largely depends on the presence or absence of fetal testicular hormones. In the absence of testicular hormones, a female type of tract will develop; in the presence of testicular hormones, a male type.

A naturally occurring example showing the effect of male hormones on the developing female reproductive tract is the freemartin in cattle. A freemartin is a genetically female calf whose reproductive tract has become modified *in utero* towards the male form. The criteria necessary for this to take place are: a twin pregnancy, one of the embryos being female and the other male; and the establishment of an anastomosis between the chorionic blood vessels of the two embryos. The changes occur only in the female member of a pair of fetuses meeting these conditions and do not develop in the absence of a vascular anastomosis. The explanation of the phenomenon, that hormones from the male reach the circulation of the female and act on its developing reproductive tract, is in agreement with experimental findings described above.

A more complete understanding of the role of testicular secretions has been derived from studies of the effect of making testicular grafts into genetically female embryos, or the exposure of such embryos to androgens. Such work has shown that the masculinising effects of testicular tissue does not depend only on its presence in an embryo, but on its localisation. Masculinisation of the genital tract of a female rabbit fetus required that the testis be grafted close to the tract. Furthermore, if such a graft was made unilaterally, the masculinisation was also unilateral, although the effect extended longitudinally along the affected tract. A comparable effect follows unilateral castration of male fetuses at the appropriate time of development, when absent or incomplete masculinisation of the genital tract on the castrated side occurs. A similar localised response follows the implantation of a crystal of testosterone into a zone adjacent to the urogenital ridge of a female fetus, resulting in persistence of the complete Wolffian duct system, although development of the Müllerian ducts is not inhibited.

Fetal decapitation has already been mentioned in relation to studies of fetal pituitary activity. If performed in male rabbit fetuses the signs of feminisation which follow are found in the external genitalia, that is in those structures which lie furthest away from the testes. The effect can be prevented by the administration of gonadotropic hormone to the fetuses, which suggests that it is due to a partial testicular deficiency. But caution must be exercised in the extrapolation of the results of animal studies from one species to another even within mammals, since decapitation of fetal rats at any equivalent stage did not prevent development of a male genital tract. It would therefore be unwise to assume that the pituitary and testes of human fetuses have a role precisely similar to that in the few mammalian species studied experimentally, although there is little doubt that the general relationship between testis and differentiation of the genital tract, and particularly the external genitalia, does apply. The time scale of development of human fetuses and of many larger mammals is greatly extended compared with rats and rabbits. If anatomical stages of the development of the reproductive tracts are compared, then the critical stages in the rabbit which were noted in relation to the effect of fetal castration, namely days 20-24, correspond to CR lengths of human fetuses of about 30-50 mm occupying in time something like the first half of the third month of pregnancy.

Histochemical studies have shown that the appropriate enzymes for steroid hormone metabolism are present in human testis from about the 30 mm stage, and human fetal testicular tissue (mostly taken at somewhat later stages of development) has been shown to synthesise androgenic steroids. Yet male human anencephalic fetuses which lack pituitaries, or in which there appears to be a gross disturbance of normal hypothalamo-pituitary relationships, still have normal male genital tracts, although both reduction in testicular interstitial cells and reduced penile growth at birth has been reported in such fetuses. Perhaps the presumed impairment of pituitary activity in these fetuses only affected fetal testicular secretion of androgens after the critical phase of differentiation of male genital tracts.

Antiandrogens

The administration of the antiandrogen cyproterone acetate has allowed another kind of approach to the study of those aspects of development which are androgen-dependent during fetal life. The drug was given to adult pregnant rats at varying times during pregnancy in order to establish the precise date at which fetal gonadal development could be affected. In general it was found that the following were androgen-dependent:

(a) Stabilization of Wolffian duct (i.e. future development of vas deferens).
(b) Differentiation of male accessory glands.
(c) Development of male external genitalia.
(d) Non-development of vagina in the male.

The following were not considered to be androgen-dependent:

(a) Regression of Müllerian duct.

(b) Descent of testis.

(c) Differentiation of gonad to testis.

Viewed overall, it seems clear that in mammals generally, including man, the fetal testis produces hormones which are essential for the normal differentiation of a male reproductive tract, but that the early differentiation of the indifferent gonad to form a testis is brought about by some influences associated with the Y chromosome. The process is not however a simple one of androgens acting on an undifferentiated system, since other factors seem to be concerned in the regression of the Müllerian ducts; whether or not some unidentified hormone is responsible for this effect is uncertain. Experimental studies clearly indicate that malfunction of fetal testes at a critical stage of sexual differentiation can be associated with failure of normal differentiation of male reproductive organs in genetically male fetuses, and hence with some degree of feminisation or pseudo-hermaphroditism. The effect of androgenic steroids on the undifferentiated tracts, whether genetically male or female, also raises the question of the influence of maternal steroids, whether produced endogenously or administered, which might cross the placenta and bring about masculinisation of female fetuses. Experimental administration of androgens to pregnant mammals does have such results. In humans certain steroids, notably some "progestins", exert androgenic effects, and some degree of masculinisation of female infants whose mothers took such substances has been reported. In view of the interrelationships of various steroids (see chapter 1) it is clearly not always easy to be certain that a given steroid compound is free of the danger of transplacental effects which, if exerted at a critical stage, could severely disrupt the normal embryogenesis of female infants.

In the light of these facts an oral contraceptive is contraindicated if there is any possibility of pregnancy, and it can readily be seen that a situation might arise where a woman could ask her physician to prescribe an oral contraceptive without realising that she is already pregnant. The simple solution is to ensure that the drug is taken, as it should be, from day 5 of a period. Similarly, an intrauterine contraceptive device is best inserted during the latter part of menstrual flow. Until recently, there were steroid preparations which could be used as 'pregnancy tests' in the sense that if given to a woman complaining of amenorrhoea they would produce withdrawal bleeding after say six days treatment only if she were not pregnant. This practice has fallen into disrepute for fear of damage to the fetus.

Feminisation of male fetuses under the influence of an excess of oestrogens seems to be a less likely phenomenon, although it occurs to varying degrees after the administration of oestrogens to pregnant animals. As regards humans, there seems to be little evidence that such effects are of much significance. Unless prolonged excessive levels of oestrogenic steroids are maintained in the fetal blood, the dominant androgenic influence of testicular secretions in male fetuses prevails. The fetal testicular interstitial cells are perhaps stimulated to secrete androgens by the circulating HCG.

FETAL ADRENAL GLANDS

Development

The adrenal or suprarenal glands are made up of an outer cortex and an inner medulla, each of which develops from a different source. The cortex develops from mesothelial cells which penetrate the vascular mesenchyme of the dorsal wall of the coelomic cavity, close to the dorsal mesentery. In man the earliest proliferation of cells forms the provisional or fetal cortex, but a second proliferation soon follows and gives rise to an outer zone of cells which forms the definitive or permanent cortex. The fetal cortex constitutes the major part of the adrenal glands in the pre-natal period, and during this time the glands are relatively much larger than later in life. The fetal cortex begins to involute towards the end of pregnancy, and increasingly rapidly in the first weeks after birth, leading to an absolute decrease in the adrenals to about half their weight at birth. During this period the permanent cortex enlarges and develops three distinct zones (Fig. 18). The outer one lying immediately beneath the fibrous capsule of the gland is the zona glomerulosa. The cells of this zone are arranged in arcades, the curved aspect of the arcades abutting on the capsule. Internally the zona glomerulosa gives way to the zona fasciculata, characterised by radially arranged columns of large cells between which run capillaries. The deepest zone of the cortex is the zona reticularis, where the cells are smaller than in the zona fasciculata and are arranged in irregular cords. Ultrastructurally the cells of the z. glomerulosa show a poorly developed smooth endoplasmic reticulum; this is well developed in cells of the z. fasciculata, has a tubular arrangement, and increases in amount in secretory activity. These cells also contain prominent round or oval mitochondria and numerous lipid granules which reach a size up to about 3.0 μm. Cells of the reticularis resemble those of the fasciculata, but dense lysosomal bodies occur more frequently.

The medulla of the adrenal is formed from neuro-ectodermal cells which migrate ventrally from the neural tube and crest to penetrate the cortical mass. These cells, which are part of the chromaffin system, become innervated by pre-ganglionic nerve fibres of the sympathetic system.

Function

Growth and secretion of the permanent cortex of the adrenal are under the influence of ACTH secreted by the adenohypophysis. The effect of this tropic hormone is exerted mainly on the inner two zones, the zona fasciculata and the zona reticularis; the zona glomerulosa seems less dependent on it, and undergoes less atrophy after hypophysectomy than the other two. The zona

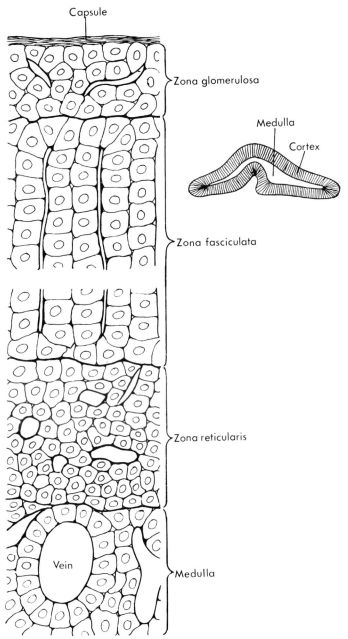

Fig. 18. Diagrams to show (top right) the naked eye and (left) microscopic appearances of sections through the human adrenal gland.

glomerulosa secretes mineralocorticoids, the chief of which is aldosterone. These act on the renal tubules bringing about the reabsorption of sodium and excretion of potassium. The two inner zones secrete a number of glucocorticoids, among which are cortisol and corticosterone, which act mainly on the metabolism of carbohydrate, protein and lipid. The cortex also secretes sex hormones, but normally only dehydroepiandrosterone in appreciable quantities. The secretion of glucocorticoids and sex hormones is dependent on ACTH.

The adrenal medulla is not under pituitary control, and the secretion of adrenaline and noradrenaline from two distinct types of medullary cell is brought about by direct stimulation of the secretory cells by sympathetic nerve fibres, which are the equivalent of preganglionic fibres. The medullary cells derived from neural ectoderm are embryologically equivalent to sympathetic ganglion cells.

The function of the fetal cortex has been difficult to elucidate since many species of animal, including those commonly available for experimental studies, do not develop this in a form comparable to that in the human. The indications are that it secretes conjugated androgens, which are transformed by the placenta into active androgens and oestrogens. The fetal cortex, like the permanent one which replaces it, appears to be largely under the control of ACTH secreted by the adenohypophysis. Anencephalic fetuses in which the pituitary has failed to develop have small adrenal glands and no fetal cortex, and hypophysectomy (by decapitation *in utero*) results in its atrophy while intact litter mates show cortices of normal size. Administration of ACTH to hypophysectomised fetuses prevents the atrophy, indicating that it is due to lack of this pituitary factor. Furthermore, a feedback mechanism of adrenal corticosteroids on the anterior pituitary, such as is known to act post-natally, also appears to be in operation *in utero,* since the administration of excessive amounts of adrenocortical hormones to intact fetuses results in atrophy of the adrenal cortex, indicating a diminished output of ACTH from the pituitary. The existence of such a feedback system has been confirmed by removal of one adrenal gland from a fetus. This results in a fall in the blood level of adrenocortical hormones and a resultant diminution of their negative feedback effect on the pituitary, which responds by an increased output of ACTH. The remaining adrenal cortex then undergoes compensatory hypertrophy.

Absence of the pituitary does not seem to result in a total loss of differentiation of the adrenal cortex, but rather in a much reduced state of differentiation. As with the gonads the effect of hypophysectomy varies according to the stage of development at which it is performed. Studies on rats and rabbits suggest that there is a critical stage during late fetal life at which the pituitary influence on cortical differentiation and cortical secretion is greatest. After this the cortex enters a relatively inactive stage; hypophysectomy of fetal rabbits during the late phase of development (26 days) had no effect on the adrenals when they were compared with control fetuses at 29 days.

The fetal adrenal cortex is fully capable of synthesising a number of steroid hormones, and evidence for this is available for larger mammals such as the sheep as well as for rats and rabbits. The full extent of the role played by these steroids in fetal growth and metabolism is not clear. One marked effect is on the deposition of glycogen in the liver and in the heart. The amount of glycogen in the liver increases suddenly in late fetal life, at the 19th day in rats and the 25th day in rabbits, and hypophysectomy (by decapitation) prior to this time results in considerably less glycogen deposition. In rats, the administration of corticosteroids restored the amount deposited to normal, but in rabbits the administration of corticosteroids proved ineffective in increasing glycogen storage in fetuses decapitated on day 26. This is another example of species differences in relation to the precise effects of hormones on metabolic processes, although the differences may be only of degree and of timing. In rabbits the induction of glycogen storage by adrenocorticoids seems to depend on a synergistic effect of some other factor acting on the liver at the same time. Storage took place in fetal rabbits decapitated on day 23 under the influence of several different agents, including extracts of rat (but not rabbit) placenta, prolactin and growth hormone. The simultaneous administration of corticoids with these substances was not always necessary for glycogen to be accumulated.

In considering the importance of fetal adrenal cortical secretion, as indeed other fetal endocrines, maternal influence by the transplacental transfer of hormones must be taken into account, since maternal adrenal cortical hormones can cross the placenta and act in the fetus. For example the glycogen stores of the liver of fetuses decapitated *in utero* were reduced to about 60% of normal in fetuses with intact mothers; but with adrenal-ectomised mothers the reduction was greater, to about 15%. Furthermore, cortisone reversed this effect whether it was administered to the fetus or to the mother.

A similar transplacental effect is observed when a pregnant rat is adrenalectomised: the operation is followed by hypertrophy of the fetal adrenals. The basis of this is that the loss of maternal adrenocortical hormones removes the possibility of maternal → fetal placental transfer of cortical hormones, but a fetal → maternal transfer can occur. This will result in a lowered fetal blood level of corticosteroids, a fall in the negative feedback effect on the fetal pituitary, an increase in fetal ACTH secretion and hypertrophy of the fetal adrenals. Conversely, diminished growth of fetal adrenal glands has been found when the mother had been treated with corticosteroids.

Involvement of the hypothalamo-hypophysial-adrenal axis in fetal adrenal activity is not surprising since the hypothalamus, which exerts a major influence on the postnatal pituitary, is also active during at any rate the later stages of fetal life. Anencephalic human fetuses in which there is disruption of normal hypothalamo-hypophysial relationships have adrenals of smaller size than normal and secrete appreciably smaller amounts of adrenocorti-costeroids. The involvement of the hypothalamus in the effects of fetal decapitation have also been shown by encephalectomy of rat fetuses, that is the removal of the brain including the hypothalamus but leaving the pituitary gland in place. This type of operation results in a reduction in size of the adrenals similar to that which follows removal of the whole head, and indicates a loss of ACTH presumably consequent to the loss of hypothalamic CRF.

DEVELOPMENTAL ANOMALIES

Congenital adrenal hyperplasia: the adrenogenital syndrome

Adrenal virilising hyperplasia is a rare pathological condition which illustrates some aspects of fetal pituitary-adrenal activity as well as endocrine influences on the development of the reproductive organs. Various types of this have been described; typically, a genetically female infant is born with a lesser or greater degree of masculinisation of the reproductive organs, particularly the external genitalia. This is a form of pseudo-hermaphroditism.

Anatomically, such an infant has external reproductive organs which appear male rather than female. The labio-scrotal folds have fused and the clitoris is enlarged to resemble a penis. No testes are present. The urethra may open at the base of the apparent penis; rarely a penile urethra may be formed. Secondary sex characteristics, notably pubic and axillary hair, may begin to appear within a few years of birth. Internally, such individuals show ill-developed female reproductive organs of Müllerian origin, while, as in normal females, Wolffian derivatives have atrophied. Ovaries are present, but ovulation does not occur; a uterus and vagina are present, the latter communicating with the urethra. The adrenal glands are greatly enlarged.

The condition may develop in fetal life, when the anatomical changes will be most marked, or may occur with varying degrees of severity at some time after birth. Adrenal hyperplasia also occurs in genetically male children; in these the genitalia are typically male, but the penis reaches adult size at an early age, and again sexual hair develops prematurely. Testes are present, but usually remain small and fail to show normal spermatogenesis. Children of either sex with this condition grow more rapidly than normal in their early years, but epiphyseal closure is early and they do not reach normal adult height.

The essential factor underlying congenital adrenal hyperplasia is an enzymatic defect of the adrenal cortices. The synthetic pathway of cortisone, in a simplified form, is:

Acetate→ cholesterol→ pregnenolone→progesterone→ 17-hydroxyprogesterone
→ deoxyhydrocortisone → hydrocortisone

The initial formation of pregnenolone is under the influence of ACTH; at each subsequent step a specific enzyme (hydroxylase dehydrogenase) is needed.

The biochemical condition found depends on the particular enzyme which is lacking, and therefore on the site of the block in the synthetic process. A deficiency of cortisone however means that the normal negative feedback effect on the secretion of ACTH is lacking, and this tropic hormone is secreted in excessive amounts, so that the adrenal cortex becomes hyperplastic. The excessive ACTH also causes the abnormal production of large amounts of pregnenolone and progesterone, which are converted to androgen; this, in abnormally large amounts, brings about virilisation, despite the presence of excessive amounts of oestrogenic steroids.

Hermaphroditism and ovotestes

Many lower vertebrates including cyclostomes and other fishes pass through a phase of normal but rudimentary hermaphroditism during which the gonads for a time contain both male and female germ cells. Usually they develop into testis or ovary, but uncommonly functional gonadal tissue of both sexes may persist into adult life. Some species, including many teleost fish show another type of hermaphroditism in which a spontaneous change from one sex (usually morphologically female with ovaries) to male with testes occurs. Experimentally true sex reversal has been achieved in female fighting fish by ovariectomy, which resulted in some females growing testes and assuming male characteristics. Following treatment of female fish with testosterone during pregnancy and exposure of the young to this hormone after birth, all the young that matured were male.

Ovotestes occur in reptiles; in amphibia testicular spermatic tubules commonly contain oocytes, and treatment of genetic males with oestrogen during development inhibits development of the medulla of the gonad and ovaries develop. Even mammals may pass through a stage of incipient hermaphroditism, and in mice for example the testes show a rudimentary and transient cortex.

Chromosomal disorders

In determining the sex of an individual, where there is some ambiguity, it is customary to examine cells from a buccal smear for chromatin and to analyse chromosomes to establish the karyotype.

Some 30% of the nuclei of cells from normal females show a special mass of chromatin near the nuclear membrane, and the individual is said to be chromatin positive. However, chromatin positive does not imply "female", just as chromatin negative (the usual condition in the male) does not strictly imply that the person is male. Individuals are, therefore, spoken of as chromatin positive or negative (with the thought that normal males are generally chromatin negative since very few of their cells can be found to contain the separate chromatin mass or 'Barr Body').

The establishment of the karyotype of an individual is now a routine procedure and any extra X or Y chromosomes may be readily detected.

Abnormalities of the Male Phenotype

Karyotype 47,XXY—chromatin positive Klinefelter's syndrome—occurs in 1 in 700 male births and may not manifest itself in signs or symptoms until puberty. However, small genitalia, undescended testicles and hypospadias may be noted, while the extra sex chromosome tends to lead to diminished intelligence. With deficient androgen secretion, puberty may be abnormal, sterility is the rule, but potency may remain. The lack of androgen appears to be correlated with decrease in aggression and small gonads.

Further karyotype abnormalities are known, notably:

Karyotypes 48,XXYY and 49,XXXXY, the extra X chromosome leading to mental deficiency.

Karyotype 46,XX in males giving a picture of Klinefelter's syndrome with a female karyotype.

Male Turner's Sydrome. These cases are phenotypically male but possess somatic abnormalities associated with Turner's syndrome (see below).

Treatment with androgens is of benefit to many cases of male chromosome abnormality, and variable degrees of sexual maturity and positive metabolic effects result.

Abnormalities of the Female Phenotype

Among these is Turner's Syndrome (ovarian dysgenesis), in which the patient is usually chromatin negative with karyotype 45,XO. There is diminished sexual development, a streaky non-functional "gonad", webbing of the neck and shortness of stature. Associated cardio-vascular abnormalities, especially coarctation of the aorta, have been noted. Another chromosomal abnormality is karyotype 47,XXX. In this there may be normal ovarian development but the subject tends to be tall and less intelligent. The addition of further X chromosomes leads to further mental deterioration.

The main problems of ovarian dysgenesis, sexual immaturity, amenorrhoea and shortness of stature are generally treated with cyclical oestrogen/progesterone therapy but care must be taken to avoid the possible complication of early fusion of epiphyses in an already small patient, and the known side effects of oestrogens (cf. patients taking the oral contraceptive) must be borne in mind in a patient taking oestrogen over a long time-span.

Failure of gonadal development

Cases of pure gonadal dysgenesis are found associated with 46,XX karyotype. Here puberty will be affected according to the degree of development of the gonad. In general the woman will have ovarian malfunction with raised gonadotropin and low oestrogen levels. Pure gonadal dysgenesis also occurs with 47,XXY karyotype. Here there is danger of gonadal development along the masculine line with the potentiality for a metastasising seminoma. These patients have female external genitalia and in addition they have a uterus. This condition is to be distinguished from that of testicular feminisation where the patient is superficially female (with female external genitalia) but lacks a uterus and has male gonads. It is likely that the tissues do not respond to androgens in the normal way. In cases of 46,XY pure gonadal dysgenesis who have been raised as girls and in testicular feminisation, it is customary to remove the gonads for fear of later malignant change. Hormonal treatment results in rearing as a female.

Cases of interdeterminate sex

A number of cases occur in which the phenotype is indeterminate and the external genitalia may be intermediate in development. The procedure is to conduct a careful clinical examination, perform a buccal smear, determine the karyotype and to exclude congenital adrenal hyperplasia (hormonal investigations may be of considerable value here).

True hermaphroditism is rare, but the following categories exist:
(a) lateral: there is an ovary on one side and a testis on the other.
(b) unilateral: there is an ovary or testis on one side but an *ovotestis* on the other.
(c) bilateral: there is an ovotestis on both sides.

These cases are considered to be whole body chimeras, being composed of a mixture of 46,XX and 46,XY cells. This might come about by fertilisation by two sperms, one fertilising the ovum and the other its second polar body; alternatively, fusion of dizygotic twins at an early stage may result in the chimera.

7

Reproduction in the Male

The male reproductive system

The male genital system consists of the two testes and their ducts, several accessory glands and the penis. As already considered in chapter 6, male and female systems have early embryological features in common, while the anatomy of the male system, particularly the external genitalia, shows essentially a further development from the early indeterminate form which the female genitalia still resemble. Such development is influenced by male hormones, and imbalance of these at certain stages of development can result in varying degrees of pseudo-hermaphroditism (see p. 82).

Functionally, the testes have in common with the ovaries a dependence on endocrine (gonadotropic) control, pre-pubertal immaturity and a dual role of both producing the germ cells and acting as glands of internal secretion. Both the ovaries and testes descend during fetal life from their original dorsal abdominal position, and carry with them their blood supply and lymphatic drainage. The ovaries normally descend only into the upper part of the "true" pelvis, while the position taken by the testes varies in different species. In some such as elephants the testes remain permanently high up in the abdominal cavity adjacent to the caudal poles of the kidney, but in many species they lie outside the abdominal cavity in the inguinal or perineal region as in most rodents, or in the scrotum as in most primates including man. The testes of some seasonally breeding mammals descend into the scrotum only during the breeding season, at other times lying within the abdominal cavity, spermatogenesis not taking place.

Descent of the testes in man occurs during fetal life, and they have usually passed through the inguinal canals to lie in the scrotum by the time of birth. In man and other mammals with scrotal testes the slightly lower temperature of the scrotum compared with that of the abdominal cavity seems to be essential for the occurrence of normal spermatogenesis, and undescended human testes do not produce mature spermatozoa, although they are capable of secreting androgens. They are also particularly susceptible to malignant change, and in view of this surgical removal of a testis that cannot be brought down is commonly advised.

The human testes are somewhat flattened egg-shaped structures, measuring about 4.5 cm in length, 2.5 cm in breadth and 3 cm in depth. Each is in close contact, indeed in continuity, with the epididymis, a long coiled part of the duct system of the testis, which forms a semi-lunar body along its posterolateral border. Each testis is made up of some 200-300 lobules, each of which contains one or more convoluted seminiferous tubules which if dissected free may extend to a length of about 70 cm. The lobules are defined by incomplete septa of connective tissue which subdivide the body of the testis and are continuous with a posterior thickening of the capsule, the mediastinum (Fig. 13c). The capsule which encloses the organ is of tough white fibrous tissue, and is called the tunica albuginea.

The seminiferous tubules constitute the part of the testis producing the male sperm cells, spermatozoa; the tubules run towards the mediastinum testis and open into straight tubules (tubuli recti) which lead to a network of ducts called the rete. From this a dozen or so efferent ductules pass to the head (rostral part) of the epididymis and join its duct, a single tubule several metres in length coiled within the epididymis. This leads inferiorly into the vas deferens, a thick walled duct which carries the spermatozoa from the testis to the ejaculatory duct in the prostate gland and thence into the prostatic urethra.

The seminiferous tubules consist of an outer layer of dense fibrous tissue and a basement membrane enclosing a stratified germinal epithelium. The cell line within this epithelium leading to the development of spermatozoa is (Fig. 19):

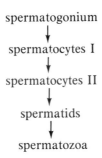

The spermatogonia, the stem cells, lie deeply in the tubal epithelium against the basal lamina. During active spermatogenesis these cells divide mitotically. The daughter cells may either divide to form more stem cells or, after increasing in size, divide to form two primary spermatocytes. These still have the diploid number of chromosomes (see p. 49), in man 22 pairs of autosomes and a pair of sex chromosomes. Each primary spermatocyte undergoes the first meiotic or reduction division to produce a pair of secondary spermatocytes each having only 23 chromosomes. These have a relatively short existence and soon divide to give two spermatids, which contain 23 chromosomes, each with only one chromatid. The formation of the spermatids marks the end of spermatogenesis. The final stages, in which the spermatids are transformed

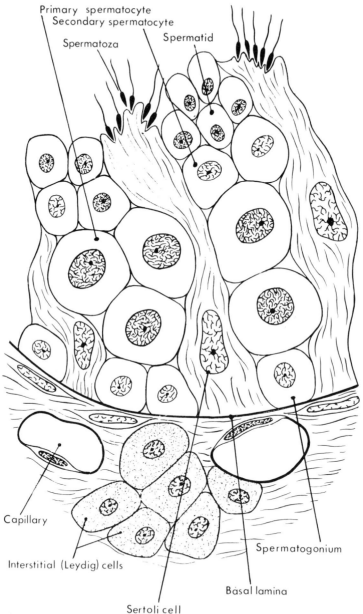

Fig. 19. Diagram to show the microscopic structure of the testis. Part of one seminiferous tubule and an interstitial zone are shown. Tight junctions which occur between Sertoli cells, are not illustrated.

without further division into spermatozoa, constitute spermiogenesis. The whole process, from spermatogonia to spermatozoa extends over about 64 days in man.

Lying among the germinal cells are large irregularly shaped cells of another type, called Sertoli cells, which extend from the basement membrane of the tubule to the luminal border of the epithelium. These are difficult to define in histological preparations due to their irregular outline and close association with germinal cells. Their apical parts are often invaginated by the heads of spermatozoa, a relationship which gave rise to the suggestion that the Sertoli cells might play a part in their nutrition. Electron microscopy has clarified some aspects of the relationship of Sertoli cells to other elements of the seminiferous tubules and confirmed their intimate relationship to cells of the germinal epithelium, which lie within depressions or pockets in their surface. Adjacent Sertoli cells are joined by tight junctional membranes which form a barrier across the intercellular spaces and, as shown by the impermeability of these junctions to substances such as colloidal lanthium nitrate, prevent the passage of large molecules. Extending as they do from the basement membrane of a tubule to its lumen, the cytoplasm of the Sertoli cells joins the perivascular extratubular space to the tubular lumen in a way somewhat similar to ependymal cells of the central nervous system. They are thus placed in such a way that they could act as a selective barrier to the passage of substances in either direction, and it has been suggested that they may guard against the passage of some materials into the seminiferous tubules and protect the germinal epithelium from noxious substances. They are know to be phagocytic, and they ingest and break down fragments of spermatids. Their possible role as nutrient cells for elements of the germinal epithelium and for spermatozoa is not yet proved. It has been suggested that the Sertoli cells secrete androgen, possibly testosterone, and the secretion of oestrogen has also been attributed to them (see below).

Scanty vascular connective tissue surrounds the seminiferous tubules; this is increased in amount in many areas, forming intertubular islands of tissue in which lie small clumps of rounded or polygonal cells. These are the interstitial or Leydig cells. They are steroid-secreting endocrine cells and produce the hormone testosterone under the control of the pituitary gonadotropin LH (see below). Electron microscopy shows that the cytoplasm of these cells contains abundant smooth endoplasmic reticulum in the form of tubules, flattened cisternae and annulate lamellae. Lipid droplets are numerous. In human interstitial cells is found a characteristic polygonal body with sharp edges and a regular internal structure; this is the proteinaceous crystalloid of Reinke, whose significance is unknown.

The volume of seminal fluid ejaculated in man is usually between 2 and 6 ml. It consists of the spermatozoa and the seminal plasma, derived from the testes and the accessory glands of the reproductive tract, the seminal vesicles, prostate and bulbo-urethral glands.

The two seminal vesicles each consist of a single tube 10-15 cm long, but sacculated to form a structure about 5 cm long. Each joins with the terminal part of the vas deferens of its own side to form the ejaculatory duct, which opens into the prostatic urethra on a small swelling. The mucosal lining of the vesicles has a pseudostratified columnar epithelium and is thrown into complex folds; their walls contain smooth muscle. In cross section the terminal expanded part of the vas, the ampulla, which lies medial to the vesicle, resembles it in the complex folding of its mucosa. The ampulla differs structurally from the rest of the vas, which is a small epithelial-lined tube with a thick fibro-muscular wall. The seminal vesicles were at one time thought to serve as a store for spermatozoa, but they are essentially secretory organs, contributing to the seminal fluid globulins, vitamin C, fructose and prostaglandins.

The prostate gland, often described as being about the size of a chestnut, lies at the base of the bladder and is penetrated by the urethra and the two ejaculatory ducts. It is made up of a variable number, up to about 50, of glandular follicles which drain via a dozen or more ducts into the prostatic urethra. These secretory structures lie in a stroma consisting predominantly of smooth muscle and the whole gland is enclosed in a capsule. A midline blind diverticulum from the prostatic urethra, the prostatic utricle, runs into the prostate; it is a remnant of the paramesonephric ducts. The prostate secretes a fluid which contains acid phosphatase. It was initially thought to be the major source of seminal prostaglandins (see p. 124).

The smallest of the male accessory organs are the two bulbo-urethral glands, pea-sized structures which lie above the bulb of the penis, enclosed by fibres of the urethral sphincter muscle. The mucoid secretion of each gland drains by a duct up to about 3 cm long into the posterior part of the spongy urethra, and serves as a lubricant prior to ejaculation.

Prepubertal development

The fetal testis contains rudimentary seminiferous "tubules" although these do not have a lumen. At this time the interstitium is packed with Leydig cells similar to those which appear at puberty. These generally atrophy rapidly in the early postnatal period, and by the time the child is a few months old none are detectable. Later, during childhood, the Leydig cells are atypical in appearance, and resemble fibroblasts. They become prominent and differentiated at puberty, and in the adult testis often contain pigment and lipid material. In senility these cells are still present, although often reduced in number.

The seminiferous tubules develop slowly during childhood, and generally a lumen is present after six years. At puberty they increase in size and become more tortuous; these changes precede the growth of interstitial cells. Mitotic and meiotic activity of the germinal epithelium gradually develops, the tubular lining assumes its mature form and the Sertoli cells differentiate. By this time the lumen of the tubules occupies about one third of the cross-sectional tubular diameter.

Development of the prostate is largely postnatal. At birth there are no follicles, and the gland consists of a system of ducts embedded in stroma, with solid epithelial buds at the site of the future secretory acini. The epithelium of the ducts begins to hypertrophy at about 9-10 years by budding. This process continues until puberty, when the gland increases rapidly in size as follicles develop, and within six to twelve months has become twice as large as in the immediate pre-pubertal phase.

Testicular activity

Puberty in the male (Chapter 4) is marked by the gradual development of secondary sexual characteristics—the growth of pubic, axillary and body hair, the breaking of the voice associated with growth changes in the larynx, the achievement of male bodily form and the development of sexual activity. The penis and testes enlarge, spermatogenesis begins, output of testicular androgens gradually increases and the accessory reproductive glands become actively secretory. Libido increases, and ejaculation can be achieved. The changes are not sudden, but rather take the form of gradual growth and development, culminating for the gonads and accessory reproductive glands in full secretory activity.

Reproductive cycles comparable with those of the female do not occur in the human male, but many species of mammal are seasonal breeders, for example the ferret, shrew and hedgehog; in such species males as well as females exhibit a limited annual period of reproductive activity. During this phase, which is normally coincident with the time when the females are undergoing oestrous cycles, androgen secretion is maximal, the accessory reproductive glands under androgenic stimulation are highly active and spermatogenesis is taking place in the testes. Outside the breeding season the testes are relatively inactive and spermatogenesis is absent. As already described, the testes in some species remain intra-abdominal for much of the year and only descend into the scrotal sac at the breeding season.

Man in common with some other mammalian species is a continuous breeder and spermatogenesis, together with secretion of androgens and consequent activity of accessory reproductive glands, continues throughout the year. Hence fertile mating at the appropriate stage of the female cycle can occur at any time, although this does not exclude the possibility of some seasonal influence on human reproductive activity. In males, as in females, the hypothalamo-pituitary-gonadal axis is fundamental to the reproductive process but the testes are the chief target organs for the gonadotropins. Like the ovaries, they not only produce the germ cells but also secrete sex steroids which in turn act on the accessory reproductive organs, and in the male the seminal vesicles, prostate gland and the small bulbo-urethral glands are under androgenic control. In many mammals these accessory glands are relatively much larger and more complex both structurally and functionally than in man. In the male hedgehog, for example, the reproductive organs during the mating season may constitute some 10% of the body weight.

HORMONAL CONTROL

As already described, the testes and ovaries are both largely controlled by the two adenohypophysial hormones, FSH and LH, the latter often in the male called ICSH, interstitial cell stimulating hormone, on account of its main target, the interstitial or Leydig cells. To minimise confusion the term LH is used here, even when dealing with the male.

The fact that the testis has a similar embryological derivation to that of the ovary perhaps makes it seem less surprising that both FSH and LH are essentially identical in male and female. The major difference between the two sexes is the pattern of their secretion, which is governed by the sexual differentiation of the hypothalamus. In the normal sexually mature male these two hormones seem to be secreted at a fairly constant rate, in contrast to the striking fluctuations during the menstrual cycle (p. 33).

The time and degree of response of the testes to hypophysectomy varies in different species, but in general loss of the pituitary is followed by testicular atrophy, disappearance of active spermatogenesis and atrophy of the in-terstitial cells. In man all spermatogenic cells disappear with the exception of the spermatogonia; Sertoli cells are said to persist in the hypophysectomised monkey. The loss of testicular androgens due to interstitial cell atrophy is primarily reflected in the atrophy of the accessory reproductive glands.

Studies of the recovery of spermatogenesis in hypophysectomised male human patients indicate that two types of gonadotropic hormone may be required for completion of the process. Human chorionic gonadotropin (HCG) was found to stimulate the spermatogonial phase, with the production of primary spermatocytes as well as both Sertoli and Leydig cells. Human menopausal gonadotropin (HMG) alone stimulated all phases of sperm production but less markedly the spermiogenic phase, and had a weak effect on Leydig cells. Probably both FSH and LH play a part at all phases of devel-opment of the germ cells, but completion of spermatogenesis may depend on a high LH/FSH ratio.

Despite its action in promoting spermatogenesis, lack of FSH need not necessarily result in total abolition of this activity. LH given to hypophy-sectomised adult male rats from the time of operation can maintain the whole reproductive system in a normal state. Furthermore there is now a considerable body of evidence showing that testosterone and other androgens can maintain spermatogenesis in hypophysectomised animals. Testosterone however is not a complete replacement for FSH, since the testes and the tubules in such animals are much smaller than normal, although true spermatogenesis, not simply maintenance of cells of the germinal epithelium already present, does occur. Provided an adequate amount of androgen is given, the androgen-dependent accessory glands will also be maintained in an active state but the interstitial cells, which are normally LH-maintained, atrophy.

Testicular androgen is necessary both for the completion of normal spermatogenesis and for the maturation of spermatozoa in the epididymis. It has been suggested that FSH, acting via androgen-binding protein, is responsible for the accumulation of androgen within the seminiferous tubules which is accessible to the androgen-dependent cells. Pellets of androgen implanted into the testes exert a marked stimulatory effect on tubules in their vicinity, so that the normal close physical association between the interstitial cells and the tubules might be of considerable functional importance. These secretory cells lie in areas of connective tissue related to several tubules and capillaries associated with each group of interstitial cells are supplied by branches of the testicular artery. It has been shown that in rats this blood then passes through capillaries closely related to the tubules before draining into the venous side of the circulation, an arrangement which may ensure that androgens are carried directly to the tubules from the interstitial cells.

Sertoli cells may also produce androgens, and FSH has been shown to localise on them. If they do produce androgen this raises the problem of the relationship between the Sertoli cells and the Leydig cells. The complex structural boundary between the general epithelial lining of the seminiferous tubules and the lumina of the testicular blood and lymphatic vessels could perhaps ensure that the Leydig cell androgen did not penetrate the tubules in significant amounts. This view apparently conflicts with that set out above, that androgen from the Leydig cells is an important factor in spermatogenesis. The answer may be that the Sertoli and the Leydig cells play a complementary role.

Feedback

It is generally accepted that FSH and LH have primarily different targets in the testis, LH acting on the interstitial Leydig cells and bringing about the secretion of testosterone, FSH acting on the seminiferous tubules and promoting spermatogenesis. As far as the LH-Leydig cell relationship goes, there seems to be a target organ-anterior pituitary negative feedback system in which an increased output of testosterone leading to a raised plasma level acts on the hypothalamo-pituitary complex to reduce the output of LH, and thus that of testosterone. Further evidence for the role of LH stems from the demonstration that radioactive LH is localised in Leydig cells.

A similar kind of mechanism seems to operate for the secretion of FSH, but precise details of the kind of feedback are uncertain. FSH acts on the seminiferous tubules and brings about an increase in testicular size due to tubular growth; but it appears to have no appreciable action on the Leydig cells, although a synergic action with LH has been suggested.

In men with generalised testicular damage affecting both seminiferous tubules and Leydig cells, there is an increased secretion of both FSH and LH. If however the tubules are severely damaged but the Leydig cells spared, then the secretion of LH remains at a normal level. Furthermore testosterone as well as oestrogens can suppress the secretion of FSH, although its effect on the secretion of LH is more marked. Testicular androgens seem unlikely to play the major role in any feedback control of FSH secretion. It has been proposed that a factor secreted by the germinal epithelium, "inhibin", acts in this way. A further hypothesis is that utilisation of FSH by the germinal epithelium controls the secretion of the hormone.

8

Infertility

Infertility may result from a variety of causes, including primary chromosomal disorders considered in chapter 6, but this discussion is limited to infertility stemming directly from the endocrine mechanisms underlying normal reproductive activity.

The role of hormones in the normal development of the reproductive system has already been discussed (p. 82) and it is clear that conditions such as that associated with congenital adrenal hyperplasia may induce abnormalities both in the development of the reproductive organs and in the establishment of the endocrine pattern which underlies normal reproductive processes. Similarly a variety of hormonal derangements in the period of growth and development leading to puberty interfere with the onset of fertility at the expected time. The main aspect considered here however is that of failure of ovulation associated with deficiencies in endocrine secretion, without any detailed discussion of the precise causes of such endocrine deficiency.

FEMALE INFERTILITY

The various levels of activity and hormonal events which bring about ovulation have already been considered in earlier chapters. To summarise briefly, the salient features are the secretion of FSH and LH by the pars distalis of the pituitary gland in an appropriate time-quantity pattern to bring about effective stimulation of one or more ovarian follicles to the point of rupture. This secretion is under the control of the hypothalamic releasing hormone, LH/FSH-RH, in the portal blood. The way in which a single hypothalamic hormone acts on two specific types of cell, inducing a differential pattern of secretion of FSH and LH, is not entirely clear. It probably involves different time scales of sensitivity of the two types of gonadotropic cell (FSH- and LH-secreting) to the effects of LH/FSH-RH on synthesis, storage and release of the tropic hormones, together with modulating effects exerted by the ovarian hormones on the secretion of both the tropic and hypothalamic hormones through the various "feedback" mechanisms.

A simple way of considering the essential control of ovulatory cycles in women is to regard the mechanism as a three-tier system, consisting of the hypothalamus, the anterior pituitary and the ovaries. This is sometimes referred to as the hypothalamo-pituitary-ovarian (H-P-O) axis. Failure of ovulation can result from malfunction at any of these levels, namely:

failure of the hypothalamic elements concerned to synthesise or release LH/FSH-RH;

failure of the pituitary to react to this hormone by appropriate synthesis and/or release of the gonadotropic factors FSH and LH;

failure of the ovaries to react to the gonadotropic hormones.

Interference with the transport of the hypothalamic releasing hormone can also result in loss of gonadotropin secretion; this may result from obstruction or division of the portal venules, preventing adequate concentrations of hypothalamic hormone reaching the anterior pituitary. Furthermore, since the portal veins constitute the sole, or at any rate the major, blood supply to the anterior pituitary in man and many animals, such vascular deficiency would also be likely to result in ischaemic damage to the gland and consequent loss of secretory cells.

No matter which level of this mechanism is affected the result will be not only a lack of ovulation, but also deficient secretion of the ovarian oestrogens and progesterone. Hence normal menstrual cycles and the associated cyclical changes in the reproductive tract will not occur and the feedback effects on the hypothalamo-pituitary axis normally exerted by the ovarian hormones in the course of the normal cycle will be lacking.

The hormonal state will however differ appreciably according to whether the defect involves the two "upper levels" or the lower ovarian one. If the synthesis of hypothalamic releasing hormone is deficient, or if it is not secreted into the portal blood, there will be a diminution or total absence of secretion of the gonadotropic hormones FSH and LH from the pituitary. A similar effect will occur if the cells of the pars distalis are insensitive to the releasing hormone. In both these conditions the plasma and the urine will show a reduction in their content of gonadotropic hormones. If on the other hand the primary defect involves the ovary, and provided that the hypothalamo-pituitary complex is not itself impaired, the output of pituitary gonadotropin unrestrained by the negative feedback effect of ovarian hormones will be greater than normal, and urinary titres correspondingly increased over normal levels.

The occurrence of menstrual periods is not necessarily an indication of fertility, since anovulatory cycles do occur. The absence of menstruation however is probably associated with infertility, although not necessarily, since a woman can become pregnant after a phase of amenorrhoea without passing through a full cycle to the stage of menstrual bleeding, should the first ovum ovulated after the phase of amenorrhoea be fertilised.

General causes of hormonal infertility

It is not proposed to consider here in detail the pharmacological, pathological and other aspects of disturbances of the H-P-O axis, but rather to outline in general terms the kind of factors which may be involved.

At the level of the hypothalamus damage due to infection, tumours or injury can interfere with the synthesis of hypothalamic releasing hormones and their secretion into the blood passing through the primary plexus of the portal system. Certain drugs may act at this level and by involving neural mechanisms (decreasing the amounts of neurotransmitter substances for example) prevent the secretion of hormones. Oestrogen-progestogen combinations used as oral contraceptives also act at the level of the hypothalamus, reducing the secretion of LH/FSH-RH (see p. 114).

Infertility and amenorrhoea

Primary involvement of the pituitary gland, even if the hypothalamus is capable of normal activity, may result in a deficiency in the production of FSH and LH. This is likely to be associated with deficiencies in other tropic hormones, a pan-hypopituitarism. A total loss of tropic hormones of course follows complete surgical hypophysectomy. Pituitary tumours may be associated with variable effects on secretion of hormones, including deficiencies resulting from damage (by pressure, for example) to secretory cells. Necrosis of the anterior pituitary in Sheehan's syndrome, in which there is thrombosis of the portal venules and consequent loss of pituitary tissue with the formation of fibrous scar tissue if the individual survives long enough, may result in major or minor loss of pituitary function. Deficiencies of gonadotropic secretions are commonly apparent with a lesser degree of pituitary damage than that which affects the other tropic hormones. Uncommonly, an isolated lack of gonadotropin secretion may occur with no other deficiencies.

Instances of amenorrhoea and infertility in which there is lack of clear evidence of primary involvement of either the hypothalamus or pituitary have been classified as idiopathic, or cause unkown. This is in part due to lack of full understanding of the relationship of "higher centres" of the central nervous system to the hypothalamus. It has long been appreciated that various forms of psychological stress are associated with disturbances of the normal menstrual cycle and fertility. It is also well established that many regions of the central nervous system have neuronal connections with the hypothalamus and that hypothalamic activity (not only reproductive aspects) can be changed by the influence of these areas, which among others include the cerebral cortex and the "limbic" system. Studies with animals (not necessarily applicable to man) have shown that a variety of environmental factors such as olfactory stimuli, light and temperature, can profoundly influence reproductivity, acting ultimately via the hypothalamus (see p. 133).

Abnormalities of the ovaries, the target organs of the gonadotropic hormones, may render them unable to respond to stimulation by pituitary hormones. If the capacity of the ovaries to secrete oestrogens and progesterone is impaired, the usual feedback effects of these hormones on the hypothalamus will not operate and normal cycles will not occur. Failure of normal development of the ovaries (dysgenesis) will result in lack of ovulation. Tumours of the ovary may be associated with altered levels of secretion of the ovarian steroids and, by disturbing the normal place of the ovaries in the H-P-O axis, can give menstrual irregularities.

Amenorrhoea may be either primary, when menstruation has never occurred, or secondary, when cycles stop. Primary amenorrhoea may indicate a disturbance of the H-P-O axis which is already in being at or before the expected time of the menarche, and may be associated with gross pathological conditions of the hypothalamus, pituitary or ovaries, or with suppression of the axis by unknown causes. One factor, it has been suggested, is a failure of the hypothalamus to develop the decreased sensitivity to the feedback effects of the ovarian steroids which normally occurs at puberty (see p. 47).

The treatment of infertility naturally depends on the underlying cause. If this involves the ovaries, as in primary ovarian failure, then the administration of gonadotropic hormones will be ineffective. If however the failure lies at the level of the hypothalamo-pituitary complex, and if the ovaries are potentially able to respond to appropriate stimulation, then the administration of gonadotropin or synthetic LH/FSH-RH stands a reasonable chance of bringing about ovulation.

Treatment. Regimes to induce ovulation differ, but essentially an attempt is made to initiate the pattern of hormonal secretion characteristic of normal menstrual cycles. Some form of FSH is given to induce follicular maturation followed by LH to trigger ovulation. In the absence of synthetic FSH and LH, the acquisition of sufficient hormones to treat large numbers of patients was a problem, although pig and beef pituitaries are available from slaughterhouses and extraction of the appropriate principle is perfectly feasible. Ideally human hormones are desirable, but sufficient amounts cannot readily be obtained. Post-menopausal urine however contains an appreciable amount of FSH, while the urine of women in pregnancy contains a large amount of chorionic gonadotropin (HCG) which resembles LH in its activity. Hence these two factors can be obtained by extraction from urine.

Gonadotropic treatments for infertility have been associated with a relatively high proportion of patients with multiple pregnancies, presumably due to the unphysiological hormonal sequence and dosage which must result from the administration of exogenous gonadotropins. Normally, only a single follicle in the human ovary matures to the point of ovulation in any one cycle, and although twins are not rare (1 in 100), triplets, quadruplets and quintuplets become progressively more so. The factors which may be involved in the causation of mutliple ovulation in women are firstly overdosage with FSH, which may cause maturation of a number of follicles rather than one; secondly, extended treatment with the LH-like HCG which, by prolonging the effect normally produced by the "pre-ovulatory surge" of LH, may allow more follicles to rupture as they mature in succession; thirdly, multiple pregnancy may result from a high concentration of LH in the therapeutic agent used.

One of the difficulties of achieving the optimal dosage to procure ovulation of only one follicle seems to have been the problem of assessing precisely the level of pituitary gonadotropic activity present at the time of treatment. Women with some residual gonadotropic function may be at greater risk of multiple pregnancy than those who have none; the avoidance of conception following the first treatment with human gonadotropins might decrease the chances of multiple pregnancy.

Various attempts have been made to achieve better control over the induction of ovulation. One approach has been to use substances other than the gonadotropins already discussed; another has been to attempt to overcome the inevitable variations in the response of different women to exogenous hormones which depend, among other factors, on the residual activity of their pituitary glands and the sensitivity of their ovaries to hormonal stimulation. Jones and his colleagues (1969) attempted to produce in patients a "steady state of pituitary and ovarian quiescence" by treating patients with synthetic steroids for two months before giving gonadotropins. The authors concluded however, after consideration of their results, that although it appears on theoretical grounds that a steady state could be induced, in practice this cannot be achieved since the optimal dosage of FSH and LH for different woman will probably vary with the adequacy of each one's tonic and cyclic LH secretion. They also came to the interesting conclusion that the dose of FSH is the most critical factor and that, provided this is optimal, there is no possibility of giving too much HCG, the response to this being dependent on the condition of the FSH-stimulated ovaries. Too little FSH can still be followed by ovulation, but may result in an inadequate luteal phase; too much FSH will lead to too many mature follicles.

In all treatment of this kind a major problem is achieving the precise balance between FSH and LH which occurs in the normal cycle. If FSH acts only to stimulate growth of the follicles, while LH is necessary for the secretion of oestrogen, then the purity of the FSH (i.e. degree of freedom from contaminating LH) is of great importance. Relative lack of LH in the follicular phase of the induced cycle might well, as Jones and his colleagues point out, result in stimulation of more follicles to produce the amount of oestrogen that would have been secreted had sufficient LH been present.

A different kind of approach to the problem of balancing the dosage of "physiological" exogenous gonadotropins is the use of non-natural compounds. In the last few years a number of these have been investigated and one in particular, clomiphene citrate, has been extensively used clinically. Clomiphene is a non-steroidal triethylene derivative, which acts by stimulating the release of LH/FSH-RH and can induce ovulation, provided the pituitary gland can produce gonadotropins. A considerable rise in the output of oestrogens follows its administration.

Clomiphene is not itself oestrogenic, but appears to act as an antagonist to oestrogen. It has been suggested by Bishop that it may act by competing with endogenous oestrogen peripherally or at the level of the hypothalamus-pituitary, and in this way stimulate the production of FSH and LH. Available evidence indicates that clomiphene has some advantages over the use of exogenous gonadotropins in the treatment of infertility in that the likelihood of multiple pregnancies is less, although still greater than in normally ovulating women.

The relatively recent availability of synthetic LH/FSH-RH has made possible the clinical use of this compound in appropriate cases of infertility. Administration is followed by elevation of plasma FSH and LH, provided that the gonadotropic cells of the pituitary are capable of secretion. The hormone exerts this effect in men as well as women. Drawbacks to the clinical use of this hypothalamic hormone are its short half-life and the great dilution which necessarily occurs when it is injected into the systemic circulation compared with the concentration achieved by direct secretion into the portal blood.

Recently, infertility in some women has been found to be associated with raised blood levels of LTH, or with evidence of over-secretion of this hormone manifesting itself as galactorrhoea (inappropriate lactation). Some such patients may have normal levels of gonadotropins. A long-lasting dopamine receptor agonist, Bromocriptine, has been successfully used in treatment of this condition, resulting in a lowering of the blood levels of LTH and restoration of fertility.

MALE INFERTILITY

Normal reproductive function in the male as in the female depends on the hypothalamo-pituitary-gonadal axis. Thus there must be secretion of releasing hormone by the hypothalamus; the anterior pituitary gland must be able to respond to the hypothalamic stimuli by the release of FSH and LH (ICSH); and the testes must be able to respond to the gonadotropic hormones by spermatogenesis and the release of testicular androgens, which in turn influence the accessory reproductive glands.

Testicular insufficiency may thus be secondary to dysfunction at the higher levels of the axis. The hypothalamus may not be normally responsive to feedback effects or may simply fail to secrete releasing hormone in the usual manner into the portal blood, or the anterior pituitary itself may not respond to the hypothalamic influence by adequate secretion of the gonadotropic hormones. Such secondary testicular failure may, in summary, be due to:

isolated gonadotropin deficiency of FSH and LH; gonadotropin deficiency associated with a more general lack of pituitary hormones due to pituitary or hypothalamic disease, probably of early onset; gonadotropin deficiency of late onset.

Hypogonadism developing after puberty is associated with reduction in potency and libido with gradual regression of male secondary sexual characteristics. If the tubules alone are affected there is infertility; if the Leydig cells are involved there will be a deficiency in androgen production.

Primary hypogonadism developing before puberty is associated with eunuchoidal features, notably:

Immature genitalia: infantile penis, small soft testicles and a smooth scrotum are found.

Abnormal skeletal proportions: there is delay in closure of epiphyses, denoting immature bone age; the span is more than two inches greater than the height; there is further disproportion in that the distance from the sole of the foot to pubis is two inches greater than from the pubis to vertex.

Abnormalities in muscles, body hair and voice: muscles are fine and weaker; facial hair is soft and shaving infrequently required and axillary and pubic hair scanty; the voice is high pitched.

Hypogonadism may be classified as follows:

1. *Disease of the testis*
(a) involving tubules and interstital cells.
> Testicular agenesis.
> Mumps, bilateral torsion.
> Bilateral cryptorchidism.
> Klinefelter's syndrome (seminiferous tubule dysgenesis with chromosome abnormality).
> Reifenstein's syndrome (similar to Klinefelter's but with no chromosome abnormality).

(b) involving tubules only.
> Sertoli cell syndrome (infertility but normal secondary sexual characteristics).
> Damage due to external agents such as X-rays or certain drugs (cytotoxins).

(c) involving interstitial cells only.
> Disorders of androgen biosynthesis.
> Idiopathic failure ("male climacteric").

2. *Mechanical disorders*
> Lesions of ducts; absence of vas or seminal vesical or obstruction of epididymis or ejaculatory ducts.
> Ejaculatory dysfunction; impotence (multifactorial).

The list of causes of hypogonadism is long, but many of the conditions listed above are very rare. Determination of the underlying cause of testicular insufficiency is essential before the type of treatment is decided, since clearly it is only in those conditions in which the deficiency is essentially a hormonal one that hormonal treatment is likely to be of any value. In general, an early diagnosis of a specific deficiency will lead to help through appropriate replacement therapy. Much more common is the problem of delayed puberty. Often there is no obvious abnormality, and once the above-mentioned causes of hypogonadism have been excluded time will usually see the individual through to a late but normal puberty.

Testicular tumours

These account for up to 2% of malignant tumours in man. They are generally classified as:
1. seminoma.
2. teratoma.
3. combined seminoma and teratoma.
The above are of germinal cell origin.
4. Sertoli cell tumours.
5. Leydig cell tumours.

The germinal cell tumours tend to be malignant and often an HCG-like activity can be found in the urine/plasma of patients with these tumours. Tumours of the Sertoli or Leydig cells are not so commonly malignant and may be associated with excretion of oestrogens.

AGEING

The menopause

The greater life expectancy of the present day compared with that of earlier times means that most women, unlike females of other mammalian species, now survive for a fairly long period of infertile post-reproductive life. The total human reproductive span is however greater now than a century ago, since not only does the menarche occur at an earlier age, but the menopause is postponed by some four years to an average age of about fifty.

Just as the early years of reproductive activity are commonly marked by irregular menstrual periods and anovulatory cycles, so are the later pre-menopausal ones, which constitute the climacteric. During these years fertility wanes. The ovarian population of oocytes established in fetal life is greatly diminished, and the ovarian endocrine secretions begin to fall. The physical and often emotional changes which characterise the years of the climacteric are largely due to the changing pattern of secretion of ovarian steroids.

Failure of fertility is not an abrupt event, but usually extends over some years. Its decline during the pre-menopausal phase seems to be related to degenerative changes in the ovaries associated with age. At the time when fertility begins to wane the ovaries still contain oocytes, although their numbers are greatly reduced from the beginning of reproductive life. This reduction is due not so much to the shedding of the few hundred that may have ovulated over the fertile years, but to the great losses due to atresia. Beyond about forty years of age fewer Graafian follicles are found in human ovaries and more degenerated cystic follicles appear. Together with the occurrence of anovulatory cycles, these changes result in a marked fall in the number of functional corpora lutea and hence a diminished secretion of progesterone, while the decrease in number of large follicles in the ovaries is associated with reduced secretion of oestrogens.

Studies on animals have indicated that intrinsic ovarian failure is not the only factor of importance affecting fertility. Ovaries from old mice implanted into young are maintained in full secretory activity, and ova from old mice implanted into the uteri of young ones may develop as well as those of young animals. Ovaries of young mice transplanted in old mice, however, result in few pregnancies, although the occurrence of oestrous cycles show that the pituitary glands of the old animals are capable of normal function. On the basis of these and other studies it seems that some degree of uterine failure may play a part in the decline of fertility with age. Such failure could be the result of a primary disturbance of the pattern of hormones acting on the uterus or to some intrinsic change in the endometrium, so that it fails to undergo the appropriate changes necessary for implantation.

The major physical effects of the gradual climacteric ovarian failure are due to the resultant hormonal changes. Most are associated with a lack of oestrogen and a consquent regression of the feminine characteristics which developed during puberty. The breasts, vulva and vagina undergo atrophic changes and the thinned epithelium of the latter renders it more liable to infection. The endometrium becomes thinner and its glands atrophy; smooth muscle atrophies, and the uterus eventually becomes smaller and largely fibrous; the ovaries shrink and after the menopause contain few or no oocytes. These changes are by no means sudden but extend over some years.

As a result of the failing and irregular ovarian secretion during the climacteric, the menstrual cycles tend to become less regular and shorter. When ovulation has ceased and levels of progesterone are markedly diminished, irregular fluctuations in the output of oestrogens may give rise to oestrogen-withdrawal episodes of uterine bleeding, while the diminished levels of progesterone in "normal" periods may result in scanty menstrual flow.

Bearing in mind the feedback relationship between ovarian secretions and the anterior pituitary gland, it is clear that the latter is inevitably affected by the ovarian changes. The ovulatory surge of LH characteristic of a normal mid-cycle disappears, but the lowered amounts of oestrogen put out by the ovaries do not exert the usual negative feedback effect on the pituitary, so that plasma levels of LH rise appreciably, as do the amounts secreted in the urine.

Despite the ovarian atrophy of the post-menopausal years the ovaries continue to secrete steroid hormones up to the age of 55 or later. Before atrophy is complete a few immature follicles may respond to the elevated titres of LH, undergoing luteinisation and producing some progesterone. Subsequently lack of ovarian follicles suggests that the ovarian stroma is the main site of steroid synthesis, and pregnenolone for example can be converted there to the slightly androgenic compounds dehydroepiandrosterone and androstenedione. The adrenal cortex is also a source of androgens and in some women these may be converted to oestrone. The output of adrenal androgens in the post-menopausal years coupled with the diminution of circulating female sex steroids may result in some signs of masculinisation, such as the growth of facial hair.

The major shift in hormonal balance that occurs during the climacteric and menopause is commonly accompanied by physiological manifestations of vasomotor instability, hot flushes and periods of sweating. Emotional disturbances from irritability to depression may occur. Some of the physical and emotional disabilities may respond to treatment with ovarian hormones.

Ageing in males

Despite the popular tendency to attribute unusual behaviour in middle-aged men to "the male menopause", there is little basis for the use of such a term. In the male there is no single event comparable to the final cessation of ovarian and uterine cycles which marks the end of fertility in women. Rather, there is in general a gradual deterioration in the fertilising capacity of the ejaculate with increasing age, associated with progressive degenerative changes in the testes, such as shrinkage of the seminiferous tubules and diminution of the thickness of the epithelium. This leads ultimately to obliteration of the tubules and the testes undergo progressive fibrosis, but the course of the changes is variable and old men may still be fertile. Sertoli cells persist after the germinal elements have disappeared while the interstitial (Leydig) cells may remain in apparently normal numbers, decrease, or hypertrophy. Hence, although the output of urinary androgens in general falls steadily from the mid-twenties, appreciable quantities of androgens may persist into old age.

9

Contraceptive and Other Hormones

Normal pregnancy only results if a mature ovum is fertilised by a spermatozoon and if the endometrium is appropriately prepared for the reception of the fertilised ovum by the time it enters the uterine cavity. After ovulation the human ovum retains its capacity for fertilisation for no longer than about 6 to 24 hours, and spermatozoa in the female reproductive tract seem to achieve an optimal capacity for fertilisation only after an interval (capacitation). Thus a relatively short part of each menstrual cycle is available for the initiation of pregnancy, and this pattern forms the basis for the avoidance of pregnancy by limiting intercourse to the "safe period".

The precise time of ovulation is not however invariably predictable, and until recent years contraceptive methods relied mainly on the prevention of the passage of sperm into the uterus and tubes by the use of a mechanical barrier, a sheath for the man or diaphragm for the woman; killing the sperm within the female tract by means of a spermicidal agent; or rendering the uterus hostile to the implantation of a fertilised ovum by means of a retained intrauterine device such as a small coil or ring.

CONTRACEPTIVE STEROIDS

In 1955 Gregory Pincus reported that progesterone or the synthetic compound norethynodrel would inhibit ovulation in women when taken orally. Since that time numerous steroids, mostly synthetic, have been examined for such an effect and some have come into general use as contraceptive agents. Many of these are substances which have a progesterone-like effect and can be given the general name of progestogens. It was found that the simultaneous administration of oestrogen with a progestogen made possible consistent inhibition of ovulation using a lower dose of the latter, and combinations of oestrogen and a progestogen came into use as a long-term means of contraception. The exact pattern of dosage has been varied according to the types of steroids used; progestogens may be used alone, or a combined oestrogen-progestogen pill taken for 21 days, then stopped for 7 days, which allows a "normal" menstrual bleeding. For a time a "sequential" course was favoured, in which a higher dose of oestrogen was taken for about 15 days and followed by an oestrogen-progesterone mixture for about 5 days, followed by a pause. This regimen has been discontinued.

Mode of action

The inhibition of ovulation was the "contraceptive" attribute of progestogens which brought them into favour as a means of preventing pregnancy, but even after years of study the precise mode of action is still not clear.

As discussed in chapter 3 reproductive cycles are controlled by the hypothalamo-pituitary complex which governs both maturation of the oocyte and the secretion of ovarian hormones. The latter are largely responsible for the appropriate cyclical changes in the Fallopian tubes, uterus and vagina, but also play a major part in the control of the activity of the hypothalamus and pituitary gland by feedback mechanisms. The mode of action of the various steroids used as contraceptive agents is potentially complex. They possess to varying degrees oestrogenic and progestational properties, but in addition they or their metabolites may exert some androgenic effects. They are likely to exert feedback effects on the hypothalamus in the same way as do endogenous hormones and modify the synthesis/release of LH/FSH-RH. They might also act directly on the pituitary. In either event they would modify the output of FSH and LH. Any changes induced in the hypothalamo-pituitary complex would of course be reflected in an alteration of the normal response to hormones of the ovaries, tubes and vagina. Administered substances might also influence these organs directly and in particular might alter the character of the cervical mucus. A direct effect on the oocyte or ovum is possible but perhaps unlikely, although alteration in the state of the reproductive tract will secondarily affect the fate of the egg after ovulation.

Consideration of the possible mode of action of oral contraceptives necessitates the acceptance of a number of basic premises. Thus:

1. most of the compounds used are synthetic steroids and their action, as of any exogenous substances, is superimposed on what is normally a balanced system of endogenous hormones;

2. different compounds vary considerably in their specific activities and it is unlikely that any will influence only a single aspect of biochemical activity, or indeed that their action will be limited to the reproductive system;

3. the initial evaluation of these compounds was largely based on the results of experiments with animals. Needless to say, extrapolation of such results to women is not necessarily valid, although the development of more sensitive assay methods for the levels of the various reproductive hormones in blood has enabled a more critical evaluation of the effect of contraceptive steroids. But while an action such as the suppression of ovulation can be directly assessed in experimental animals by examination of the ovaries or by recovery of ova from the reproductive tract, only by the planned timing of a necessary laparatomy or culdoscopy can such direct criteria be applied to women, although the occurrence of a possibly unwanted pregnancy will demonstrate the failure of suppression of ovulation.

Generally oral contraceptives do suppress ovulation. The ovaries lack corpora lutea and mature Graafian follicles, and histologically resemble those of post-menopausal women. While a direct effect on the ovaries cannot be ruled out, it seems likely that their most important site of action is the hypothalamus. This is strongly suggested by the demonstration that ovulation can be induced in women under treatment with an oestrogen-progestogen preparation by the administration of either exogenous gonadotropins or LH/FSH-RH.

Progestogens given alone probably abolish the mid-cycle peak of FSH, but do not necessarily suppress early follicular growth. Derivates of 17a-hydroxy-progesterone abolish the pre-ovulatory peak of LH which is normally necessary for ovulation of an appropriately mature follicle. In low dosages such compounds do not necessarily abolish the pre-ovulatory LH surge or suppress ovulation but still prevent conception. This is probably due to an effect on the cervical mucus, which may be maintained in the condition hostile to penetration by spermatozoa which normally characterises the luteal phase of the cycle. Cyclical bleeding, not necessarily according to the timing of normal cycles, occurs not uncommonly during progestogen regimes, and probably indicates the normal hormonal cycle on which the effects of the hormone being administered are superimposed.

In normal menstrual cycles oestrogens exert a negative feedback effect on the secretion of FSH. A similar action is considered to be of primary importance for the contraceptive action of combined oestrogen-progestogen regimes, follicular growth being suppressed. In normal cycles oestrogens stimulate LH secretion and act as a stimulus for the secretory peak of LH preceding ovulation. Similary, oestrogens given in small dosage in oral contraceptives may stimulate the secretion of LH, while larger doses probably do not have this effect. When given together with progestogens, they do not stimulate the secretion of LH.

On balance it is not possible to ascribe the contraceptive effect of an oestrogen-progestogen regime to an exclusive influence on either the hypothalamus-pituitary or the ovaries. The normal delicate hormonal interplay between ovaries and pituitary must inevitably be disturbed by the introduction of exogenous steroids and an alteration in secretory activity of any one part of the pituitary-ovarian axis will induce changes in the rest. Furthermore, as already noted, inhibition of ovulation is not a prerequisite of a successful contraceptive pill, and contraception can be achieved while regular ovulation occurs.

A direct effect on the ovum, preventing fertilisation despite the presence of viable sperm, is possible if unlikely. If fertilisation should occur (normally in the Fallopian tube) then the state of the reproductive tract assumes great importance. The fertilised ovum normally remains for three days in the tube before passing into the uterus. During this time cleavage is taking place and progesterone, secreted by the corpus luteum, is completing the conditioning of the endometrium to a state at which implantation is possible. The delayed passage of the ovum through the tube is critical since, if it should enter the uterus too early, the blastocyst will be less developed and the endometrium will not have reached a sufficiently progestational condition.

Leaving aside for the moment the influence of the female reproductive tract on spermatozoa, the effects of steroids on the Fallopian tube seem to be of considerable significance for the well-being of the ovum/blastocyst. Oestrogens increase stromal growth, ciliary activity and peristalsis and stimulate the secretion of tubal fluid; these effects are manifest during the first half of the normal menstrual cycle. In rabbits and rats oestrogens have been shown to increase the speed of passage of blastocysts through the tube with the result that these degenerate and pass through the uterus without implanting. Alternatively, moderate doses of oestrogens during the post-fertilisation period may cause "tube locking" of the ova, leading to eventual degeneration during cleavage. Progesterone generally seems to reduce tubal activity, and in the luteal phase of the cycle tubal contractions are of lower amplitude, ciliary movements less and the amount of fluid diminished compared with the follicular phase.

Thus a change in the normal luteal phase activity of the tube induced by exogenous steroids could be a factor in the contraceptive action. The effect of oestrogens on tubal activity evident from experimental observations on animals can probably be assumed to apply also to the human female, and indeed appropriate (but large) doses of oestrogens taken while the ovum or blastocyst is passing through the tube act as a post-coital contraceptive.

Pregnancy cannot occur if for any reason implantation of the blastocyst into the endometrium is inhibited. The progressive endometrial changes from repair through the proliferative phase to the secretory progestational state of the normal human menstrual cycle, like the comparable changes in the mammals, are precisely correlated with the ovarian changes leading to ovulation. The luteal phase is relatively short-lived unless the ovary receives further gonadotropic stimulation from the developing chorion, signalling hormonally the beginning of pregnancy. The progestational state of the endometrium however seems to be critically related to the developmental stage of the blastocyst and any marked discrepancy between the two is likely to result in failure of implantation. Again, experimental analysis is based largely on work with animals. Growth of ova can occur outside the uterine environment, as has been shown by their culture *in vitro,* the occurrence of ectopic pregnancies or the transplantation of blastocysts to sites remote from the endometrium beneath the capsule of the kidney or the spleen. In circumstances such as these variable degrees of early developmental changes occur, but apart from rare ectopic pregnancies progression is not possible beyond a stage at which dependence on the placenta normally develops.

To return to the evidence for the necessary correspondence of what may be called the "maturity" of the ovum and that of the endometrium, this has been demonstrated by transferring blastocysts of known developmental age to host uteri of a different developmental age. In rabbits implantation does not occur unless the developmental stages of blastocyst and uterus are within one day of each other. In rats blastocysts developmentally a day ahead of the uterine cornua to which they were transferred ceased to develop until the uterine development had "caught up"; normal implantation then occurred. If rat blastocysts a day younger than the uterus were transferred however they degenerated in the same way as those whose tubal passage had been unduly accelerated.

Exogenous steroids, by influencing tubal activity, may thus throw the development of the blastocyst and endometrium out of phase, and so prevent implantation. A similar end result might equally follow a direct hormonal influence on the endometrium, resulting in an alteration of its normal growth and secretory phases. The microscopic structure of the endometrium is influenced considerably by the agents used as oral contraceptives, although the precise changes vary according to the chemical structure of the steroids involved and the pattern of their dosage; such differences seem to become less with prolonged administration. The combined pill (oestrogen and progestogen) has been reported as resulting in fairly rapid regression, the endometrium changing from a proliferative to a progestational type and progressing to a non-secretory state. The sequential type of pill resulted in marked pro-liferation followed by changes corresponding to an early secretory phase. Such endometrial changes could be in part due to a direct action of the exogenous steroids, although the induced alteration of the endogenous oestrogen-progesterone levels is likely to be the major factor. Nevertheless the possibilities of exogenous steroids acting at a number of different levels, hypothalamic-pituitary, ovarian, tubal or uterine to produce the observed changes, cannot be dismissed.

Most possible modes of action so far considered have been contraceptive effects springing from some influence of the compounds on the female germ cells—suppression of their maturation and ovulation or, should ovulation and fertilisation occur, prevention of the implantation essential for pregnancy. The induction of changes in the cervical mucus already referred to is a mechanism of a different kind. In normal cycles, at about the mid-cycle time of ovulation, the physico-chemical properties of this mucus change in response to the changing hormonal balance in a way which favours the passage of spermatozoa through the cervix to the uterine cavity. Administration of some oral contraceptive substances is associated with alterations in the character-istics of the cervical mucus similar to those which occur in the progestational phase of the cycle, when it is unfavourable for sperm penetration. Such "secretory phase" mucus is secreted in women taking the combined type of pill, but as might be expected the sequential pill (oestrogen alone followed by an oestrogen-progesterone mixture) was only associated with the latter type of cervical mucus during the time that both oestrogen and progesterone were being taken. The first half of the cycle, under oestrogenic influence, was associated with mucus of lower viscosity unlikely to provide an effective barrier to sperm.

Progestogens given alone may, in certain dosages, exert their contraceptive effect by this means, although progestational-type mucus is not necessarily associated, *per se,* with any striking fall in fertility, as shown by the administration of dydrogesterone to women (Diczfalusy, 1968).

Available evidence then does little more than indicate a number of ways involving a variety of sites in which oral contraceptives may act. Inevitably the administration of any exogenous hormones, as necessarily occurs with the use of oral contraceptives, will affect the endogenous secretions. In the case of the hormonal mechanisms underlying reproductive activity the delicate balance of oestrogen and progesterone secretion, adjusted by the feedback mechanisms acting via the hypothalamo-pituitary complex, must be modified by the administration of oestrogen and/or progestogen. Since the finer points of the normal hormonal regulation of reproduction are themselves not entirely understood, it is hardly surprising that no full explanation of the precise mode of action of the oral contraceptives can be given; hence their use at the present time must be based to a considerable extent on empirical considerations.

Effects on spermatozoa

The development of oral contraceptives has been largely directed towards producing compounds influencing aspects of reproduction associated with the ovaries. Possibilities exist of a hormonal contraceptive for the male, but the effectiveness of the progestogens in current use as contraceptive agents may depend in part on their direct or indirect modification of the capacity of spermatozoa, once they are within the female reproductive tract, to fertilise an ovum.

It has been shown, at any rate for some species of mammals, that spermatozoa can fertilise an ovum only after they have spent some hours within the female reproductive tract; freshly ejaculated sperm must apparently undergo this period of "capacitation". Capacitation may be associated with modification of the acrosome cap, involving the removal of some stabilising substance. The relevance of this in the present context is that sperm capacitation is inhibited in the luteal phase of ovarian activity and also by administered progesterone. It follows that the giving of exogenous progestogens, which mimic in various ways the effects of endogenous progesterone secreted by the corpus luteum, is likely to have a comparable effect on spermatozoa within the female tract, inhibiting their capacitation and hence exerting a contraceptive action via the spermatozoa. Such effects have been studied in detail only in animals, notably the rabbit, and it cannot be assumed that the findings can be directly applied to humans.

Antiandrogens (see p. 84) might offer another approach to male contraception. These compounds (notably Cyproterone acetate) have been used in the treatment of aberrant sexual behaviour; but their tendency to lower libido has limited their use as contraceptive agents. Research continues in the hope of combining an antiandrogen which will suppress spermatogenesis with a drug which will restore libido. One might speculate that a male contraceptive which actually increased libido would excite public interest if nothing else.

Side effects of oral contraceptives

Oestrogen/progesterone regimes or progestogens alone are undoubtedly effective as contraceptive agents, and their relative safety compared even with the low mortality associated with pregnancy is recognised. Nevertheless, their use is not without side effects. Some of these are simply undesirable, but others are potentially risks to health and even to life.

Among undesirable effects, there is commonly an increase in weight when women begin to take the pill, and about a quarter of women notice fullness and tenderness of their breasts. More worrying although less frequent is the appearance of depression, headaches and migraine. When the pill is discontinued, perhaps with the intention of becoming pregnant, there may be a phase of amenorrhoea lasting several months or even longer; this may be accompanied by galactorrhoea. More acceptable side effects are the relief of primary dysmenorrhoea and of premenstrual tension.

A realistic assessment of more serious risks is difficult, partly because of the usual problems of extrapolation from the results of animal experiments to women, but partly also because inherent dangers may only become apparent after the use of contraceptive steroids over the great part of reproductive life, thirty years or more.

Apart from their effect on the normal pituitary-ovarian hormonal regulatory system, steroids having structural and functional affinities with the normal ovarian hormones are potentially active in a number of ways which may prove to be unfavourable. The lack of knowledge of the long term effect of contraceptive steroids was raised in the 1960s, and although once again the data are derived from lower mammals, there is not doubt that oestrogens can bring about modifications in some tissues of the body. In rats they cause marked changes in pituitary cytology indicative of altered secretory activity (although these animals seem to be particularly susceptible to such compounds). Pituitary adenomas in aged rats, made up of similarly excessively secreting cells, are associated with a high incidence of mammary tumours. Studies on baboons, primates not too far removed from man, also showed that marked cytological changes in the anterior pituitary occurred under the influence of oral contraceptive agents, and persisted for some time after administration had been discontinued.

Unfortunately no comparable data is available for women, but particular attention has been paid to changes in the blood chemistry, stimulated no doubt by reports of sudden death attributed to the use of oral contraceptives. A number of metabolic changes may be associated with the use of such compounds, although many of these are effects not directly involved in contraception and their ultimate effect on the health of the subject is not known. The use of oral contraceptives is associated with an increase in serum triglycerides, increased platelet sensitivity and changes in plasma proteins. A higher incidence of thrombosis and embolism in women "on the pill" is well established. Impaired glucose tolerance may occur and this, together with raised serum lipid, could in the long term lead to atherosclerotic changes and to cardiovascular disease. A number of women show a significant increase in both systolic and diastolic blood pressure, which returns to normal when they stop taking the pill. Such patients should be advised to adopt other methods of contraception.

Other endocrine glands are also influenced by oral contraceptive compounds. Oestrogens increase the iodine and the total thyroxine concentration of the plasma; both these changes are limited to the protein-bound fraction, and there does not seem to be any alteration in the secretion of TSH. Adrenal cortical activity is also affected and the amount of transcortin, the carrier protein for corticosteroids, is increased, so that the plasma levels of the protein-bound fraction of these hormones rise; this is probably of little significance.

Evidence suggests that the oestrogen component of contraceptive mixtures is the major if not the sole agent responsible for unnecessary or undesirable effects such as those described. In view of widespread anxiety it was decided to withdraw pills with an oestrogen content of more than $100 \mu g$. For practical purposes it was found that those with $50 \mu g$ were most appreciated by patients. Attempts to still further reduce the amount of oestrogen to 30 and even $20 \mu g$ were associated with breakthrough bleeding.

The oestrogen-induced side effects stimulated interest in the possibility of using one of the "progestogen-only" contraceptive agents to the exclusion of combined preparations. As already noted, such preparations may or may not suppress the mid-cycle peak of LH which plays a major role in bringing about ovulation, but they seem to have relatively little effect on the basal secretion of this hormone throughout the cycle. Chlormadinone acetate was one such substance, but this was withdrawn when it was found to be associated with the development of breast tumours in bitches. Progestogens now in common use are the 19-nortestosterone derivatives, especially norethisterone. Taken without a break the latter has had considerable success as a contraceptive agent with apparent absence of many of the unwanted effects thought to be due to oestrogens. Together with other substances having similar properties, norethisterone commonly does not inhibit ovulation, as shown by direct observation of the ovaries and by the finding that urinary gonadotropins of individuals using this substance often conform to a normal pattern. Against its apparent considerable advantages must be set a slightly lower efficiency as a contraceptive agent, compared with an oestrogen-progestogen combination. Furthermore, since it is taken without breaks there is relatively less cycle control.

Unusually, misuse of the pill may give bizarre effects as in the case of a young woman subjected to uterine curettage because of excessive bleeding. The specimens showed what appeared to be a well differentiated primary papillary carcinoma. It came to light however that despite her virginity the girl had been taking some six pills a day three weeks out of four to "prevent pregnancy". She stopped taking the pills and the endometrium, presumably extremely hyperplastic, reverted to normal; she later had a normal pregnancy.

Clinical aspects

Elstein (1975) clearly explained that the progestogen component of the oral contraceptive may vary in potency as follows:

(a) Strongly progestogenic

(b) Having additional 'anti-oestrogenic' effects (i.e. masking the effects of oestrogen)

(c) Having some oestrogenic action.

The 19-norsteroids, of which norethisterone acetate is the commonest in use, are widely favoured because of their anti-oestrogenic effect of reducing withdrawal bleeding—the "menstrual flow" which occurs at the end of each 21-day course of the pill. Preparations containing norgestrel have a systemic anti-oestrogen effect and do not produce so much action on the genital tract or affect bleeding. In practical terms, the anti-oestrogenic progestogens are useful in women who experience heavy painful periods with excessive vaginal secretion. The more systemically acting norgestrel should suit a woman complaining of loss of libido and scanty bleeding.

The appended tables illustrate the common combined preparations and their biological potency, as well as giving a guide to changes in the type of preparation prescribed when certain side-effects occur.

Before prescribing it is well to consider the woman's menstrual history. This will aid in selection of the appropriate combination and by judicious choice may well help any existing menstrual problems. The following lists attempt to categorise women into oestrogenic or progestational types, but may be of assistance when used in combination with Tables III and IV.

Oestrogenic Type: A woman whose periods may be irregular or heavy; she has oedema, is putting on weight, experiences irritability, headaches, tiredness and premenstrual tension and mastodynia. There may be heavy mucous cervical discharge and possibly a cervical erosion.

Progestational Type: She complains of light or scanty periods, some leg and possibly abdominal cramps. Dryness in the vagina, but with a white pre-menstrual discharge. There is fullness of the breasts rather than pain, and acne with greasy skin and hair may be noted.

The oestrogen component of the combined preparation is governed by the fact that the Committee for the Safety of Drugs has decreed that no pill should contain more than 50 micrograms of ethinyloestradiol. Mestranol is said to

Table III. More Potent Combined Preparations
(adapted from Elstein, 1975)

Potency	Proprietary Name	Progestogen	Strength (mg)	Oestrogen	Strength (μg)
PROGESTOGENIC ANTI-OESTROGENIC / OESTROGENIC ANTI-OESTROGENIC	Anovlar 21	Norethisterone	4.0	Ethinyloestradiol	50
	Gynovlar 21	Norethisterone	3.0	Ethinyloestradiol	50
	Norlestrin	Norethisterone	2.5	Ethinyloestradiol	50
	Eugynon-50	*dl-Norgestrel	5.0	Ethinyloestradiol	50
	Ovran	Levonorgestrel	0.25	Ethinyloestradiol	50
	Eugynon-30	Levonorgestrel	0.25	Ethinyloestradiol	30
	Ovran-30	Levonorgestrel	0.25	Ethinyloestradiol	30
	Conova-30	Ethynodiol	2.0	Ethinyloestradiol	30
	Ovulen-50	Ethynodiol	1.0	Ethinyloestradiol	50
	Minilyn	Lynoestrenol	2.5	Ethinyloestradiol	50

*NB. dl-Norgestrel: active principle is levonorgestrel 0.25 mg.

Table IV. Less Potent Combined Preparations
(adapted from Elstein, 1975)

Potency	Proprietary Name	Progestogen	Strength (mg)	Oestrogen	Strength (μg)
OESTROGENIC & PROGESTOGENIC / ANTI-OESTROGENIC	Loestrin-20	Norethisterone	1.0	Ethinyloestradiol	20
	Microgynon-30	Levonorgestrel	0.15	Ethinyloestradiol	30
	Ovranette	Levonorgestrel	0.15	Ethinyloestradiol	30
	Demulen-50	Ethynodiol	0.5	Ethinyloestradiol	50
	Norinyl-1	Norethisterone	1.0	Ethinyloestradiol	50
	Ortho-Novin 1/50	Norethisterone	1.0	Mestranol	50
	**Norinyl 1/28	Norethisterone	1.0	Mestranol	50
	Minovlar	Norethisterone	1.0	Ethinyloestradiol	50
	**Minovlar ED	Norethisterone	1.0	Ethinyloestradiol	50
	Orlest-21	Norethisterone	1.0	Ethinyloestradiol	50
	Norimin	Norethisterone	1.0	Ethinyloestradiol	35
	Brevinor	Norethisterone	0.5	Ethinyloestradiol	35
	Ovysmen	Norethisterone	0.5	Ethinyloestradiol	30

**contains 7 placebo tablets (i.e. 28 tablets in each packet and no gap between courses).

Table V. Guide to Adjustments when Side Effects Occur

Side effect	Suggested change in potency	
	Oestrogen	Progestogen
Vomiting, nausea	decrease	no change
Headache	decrease	decrease
Tiredness, irritability, pre-menstrual tension	possibly increase	decrease
Breakthrough (mid-cycle) bleeding or spotting	increase	possibly increase
Secondary amenorrhoea	increase	increase
Scanty bleeding	increase	usually no change (but may improve with Lynestrenol 2.5 mg or Megestrol 4 mg)
Heavy bleeding	no change	increase
Breast fullness	increase	decrease
Painful breasts (mastodynia)	decrease	increase
Weight gain	decrease	decrease
Weight loss	increase	increase
Hirsutism	increase	increase
Dry vagina + coital difficulty	no change	increase
Leg cramps	decrease	decrease
Oedema	decrease	no change

Sudden swelling and pain in a limb
Allergic reaction
Rise in blood pressure
Any suggestion of liver dysfunction   stop therapy with combined oral
Migraine and visual disorders   contraceptive
Chloasma
Persistent secondary amenorrhoea

have a slightly weaker action and for this reason higher amounts than 50 micrograms appear in the formulations. Many authorities believe that there is little to choose between the two but most would agree that mestranol is less potent and it may be of use in cases where nausea, retching or vomiting, are major problems. As will be seen from Tables III and IV, the majority of manufacturers use ethinyloestradiol and attempts have been made to reduce its dosage to 35, 30 and even 20 micrograms. The problem here is that spotting and breakthrough bleeding tend to occur at such low levels, but of course more serious side-effects can be minimised.

The use of progestogen-only pills is limited by the fact that they are less successful as contraceptives. Yielding pregnancy rates of 2-10 per 100 woman years* their use must be limited to those who prefer to have a small family but would not mind another child. Women of low fertility or unable to tolerate any other form of contraception may consider their use. As already discussed, they affect the cervical mucus, increasing the natural barrier noted in the luteal phase of the cycle. The absence of an oestrogen in the preparation discounts fears of thrombo-embolism, liver dysfunction and hypertension. Many physicians prefer to use this pill during lactation and in the "waiting" period after the husband has had a vasectomy (up to three months) especially when the operation has been done because of the wife's intolerance to the combined pill. Long-acting preparations such as medroxy-progesterone give about three months contraceptive effect. The progesterone-only preparations are: Femulen (ethynodiol 0.5 mg); Micronor, Noriday (norethisterone 0.35 mg).

Post-coital contraception. Oestrogens have been of value in the role of a "post-coital" pill where unprotected intercourse may have resulted in fertilisation.

The use of 0.5-2 mg ethinyloestradiol daily for five days after coitus has prevented a possible pregnancy in several trials.

PROSTAGLANDINS

As long ago as 1930 it was reported that instillation of semen into the uterus caused either strong muscular contractions or relaxation, but at that time the active principles responsible for those effects were unknown. In 1935 von Euler showed that prostatic and seminal extracts contain a principle which acts on smooth muscle. This was given the name prostaglandin, to indicate its association with the prostate, although we now know that most of the prostaglandin in the seminal fluid comes from the seminal vesicles. Since then a number of chemically related substances of the same type have been isolated; they occur in most human tissues and are also found in body fluids. Although they are not necessarily to be regarded as true hormones, they have some hormone-like effects on the female reproductive tract and, since they have also gained some prominence as possible anti-pregnancy agents, they merit some consideration here.

---

*The term Woman Year is used in calculating Pearl's Formula for Failure Rate per Hundred Woman Years (HWY):

$$HWY = \frac{\text{Total accidental pregnancies} \times 1200}{\text{Total months of exposure}}$$

Prostaglandins are biologically active lipids which appear to act as "local" hormones. They are rapidly removed from the circulation by the lungs. Despite their ubiquity, the major human source is seminal fluid and this has been studied extensively. It is convenient to refer to seminal prostaglandins as HSF-PG and to denote pure prostaglandins as PG followed by the group letter. HSF-PG contains a mixture of prostaglandins of which the main constituents are:

PGE_1 25 $\mu g/ml$; PGE_2 23 $\mu g/ml$; PGE_3 5.5 $\mu g/ml$; PGF_1 alpha 3.6 $\mu g/ml$; PGF_2 alpha 4.4 $\mu g/ml$.

The action of prostaglandins on the uterus depends on the individual PG and on the phase of the menstrual cycle. In general, intra-vaginal instillation of HSF-PG causes an increase in uterine motility around the time of ovulation, but not at the extremes of the cycle. Contraction of the corpus uteri with relaxation of the cervix has been noted, and in addition there is a general uterine relaxation after an interval of 20-30 minutes. Pure prostaglandins such as PGE_1 or PGE_2 given intravenously cause uterine contractions regardless of the phase of the cycle, while application to strips of myometrium (*in vitro*) produces conflicting results with contraction in some species and relaxation in others. It is of interest that the action of HSF-PG is enhanced by the intravenous administration of oxytocin since the latter hormone is know to be released during female orgasm.

It has been shown, *in vitro*, that PGE inhibits the spontaneous contraction of the uterine tube while PGF stimulates it. A positive Rubin's Test, i.e. contraction of the functional sphincters at the utero-tubal junction during tubal insufflation, has been reported after intra-vaginal instillation of HSF-PG in women. The anatomy of the uterine tube is such that there is a functional sphincter at the isthmo-ampullary junction as well as at the utero-tubal junction. Any delay or arrest of the zygote at the former, the so-called "isthmic block", may result in tubal implantation and an ectopic pregnancy. This region is under adrenergic control and the only reason to implicate seminal prostaglandins rests on evidence from *in vitro* experiments which suggest that HSF-PG inhibits the ampullary part of the tube while stimulating that part nearer to the uterus.

In the rat, PGE retards ovum transport; in the rabbit transport is slightly accelerated by PGE and more strongly by PGF_2 alpha. Such an effect is not however beneficial in the rabbit which is a reflex ovulator and premature arrival of the ova in the uterus before capacitation of the spermatozoa would be counter-productive. It has, nevertheless, been suggested that similar effects might be beneficial in the human where much greater amounts of prostaglandins are present and where capacitation may be of shorter duration. Blocking with indomethacin, an anti-prostaglandin, has been shown to delay implantation in mice, and since interference with ovulation was ruled out in these experiments, it was concluded that prostaglandins act directly on the tubes, the inhibiting effect of indomethacin being reversed by administration of PGE or PGF. Histoimmunological techniques have demonstrated PGF_2 alpha in the human uterine tube and a role in normal tubal motility has been suggested.

Prostaglandins occur in endometrium and in menstrual fluid, and at the time of menustration they can be detected in peripheral blood. Intravaginal instillation has been used to induce menstruation. A role in primary dysmenorrhoea has been ascribed to prostaglandins, the reasoning being that if menstrual blood is retained in the uterus rather than being voided, prostaglandins may be absorbed through the raw surface of the endometrium and bring about a general myometrial spasm giving rise to pain. Such a theory does not accord with the observations that the uterus responds markedly to prostaglandins only at about mid-cycle.

Prostaglandins have been shown to exert several effects on the ovary, both directly and via the hypothalamo-pituitary complex. At the latter level prostaglandins can increase the secretion of LH/FSH-RH and also seem to exert a direct effect on cells of the pituitary, increasing the secretion of LH. Direct effects on the ovary may increase the production of progesterone, although high dosage suppresses it. Such data stem from studies on animals, but include studies on primate (monkey) ovaries.

A principal feature of ovarian cycles is the regression of the corpus luteum when fertilisation does not occur. In non-primates, at any rate, a local luteolytic factor produced by the endometrium seems to be involved in luteal breakdown, and one uterine horn is involved in the lysis of corpora lutea in the ovary of the same side. The lytic factor may be a prostaglandin, but its mode of action is not clear. One suggestion is that it brings about vasoconstriction of a common vein which, in rats, drains both ovary and uterus, with consequent damming up of progesterone in the ovary where the steroid exerts a lytic effect. Another possibility is that prostaglandin acts directly on the ovary, interfering in some way with the stimulus of gonado-tropin or luteotropin on the corpus luteum. In women high levels of prostaglandin can cause luteal regression late in the cycle, but there is no evidence that a uterine factor is normally involved, and ovarian prostaglandins may be the active agents.

The third way in which prostaglandins may be involved in ovarian activity is in ovulation itself. Local inhibition by injected drugs of ovarian synthesis of prostaglandins has been found to be associated with interference with ovulation in rats; but the significance of this is far from clear.

Prostaglandins E and F have been found in amniotic fluid and in the maternal circulation; during labour or spontaneous abortion the quantities are considerable. Since these substances stimulate contraction of the pregnant myometrium, they may play a part in the normal process of parturition and in abortion. The pregnant uterus is sensitive to prostaglandins given intravenously and an increase in the frequency and amplitude of uterine contractions is especially marked near term. Infusions of prostaglandins have been used to induce labour in pregnant women at term and their effect is comparable to that of oxytocin. Thus prostaglandins might normally play a role in parturition, inducing or increasing uterine contractions.

Currently there is considerable interest in prostaglandins as possible abortifacients. The regression of the corpus luteum which they can effect in monkeys and other animals could presumably cause the rejection of an implanted ovum or embryo if it occurred during a time when pregnancy was luteal-dependent (see p. 54). Intravenous infusions of prostaglandins have induced abortion in women in the early months of pregnancy, and administration by vaginal pessary has also been effective. Prostaglandins acting in the early post-ovulatory phase, either causing rapid passage of the ovum through the reproductive tract or alternatively early rejection of the blastocyst, would in their final effect differ little from those of established oral contraceptives.

Prostaglandins may also play a part in male reproductive activity. They have been shown to enhance contractile activity of isolated guinea-pig vas deferens and may have some effect on sympathetically innervated tissue — the smooth muscle of the male reproductive tract, for example. The levels of PGE in semen from 40% of a group of infertile men were significantly lower than those in semen from a group of fertile men. Understanding of the real significance of these compounds in reproductive processes is just beginning, and only further studies will show their true importance.

10

Reproduction and Environment

The breeding season of a given species is commonly associated with a particular time of year, and since the 1930s an increasing understanding has developed of the important role played by environmental factors, such as light, temperature and humidity, in determining the timing of reproductive cycles.

Light

The importance of specific environmental factors varies for different species. Light, for example, exercises a considerable influence over the timing of the onset of reproductive activity in birds and many species mate, nest and lay eggs in direct response to the increasing amounts of daylight in springtime. Experimental studies have explored the relationship between environment and reproduction and clearly shown the effects of changes in the day length or photoperiod. The gonads of a group of junco finches exposed to increasing periods of artificial illumination from October onwards had developed by the end of December to a state similar to that usually found only at the normal breeding time in the spring, but a control group of birds exposed only to daylight showed no such advance.

Light is not necessarily the dominant stimulus for all species of bird. Some, such as the zebra finches inhabiting North Western Australia with its near-equatorial climate, may breed at any season of the year in response to the increased supplies of food which follow heavy rainfall. Furthermore there is not necessarily a clear cut relationship between any single environmental factor and accelerated development of the reproductive organs. Finches exposed to extra light were more active than unexposed birds and a group kept active for some four hours a day longer than a control group showed a relative increase in the size of their gonads, even when both had been kept in identical light conditions.

The timing of reproductive activity of mammals can also be considerably influenced by day length and a variety of other environmental factors. Ferrets, which have a well-defined breeding season, have been extensively studied in relation to the effects of light. Females normally come into oestrus in the spring and, in the absence of pregnancy, remain in the state until the summer. Exposure to additional light in the form of evening illumination for some eight hours daily from the end of October onwards advances the onset of oestrus by about two months. Males respond in a comparable way with accelerated testicular development and spermatogenesis. Other species, such as many kinds of sheep, respond to diminishing light and commonly breed in Britain in the latter part of the year, although this pattern can be modified by other factors.

Temperature

In some mammalian and non-mammalian species physical stimuli other than light are of particular influence. The ground-squirrel of North America becomes reproductively active in response to a lowered environmental temperature, and the warm season of the year is associated with gonadal inactivity.

The necessity for the temperature of the testes of some mammals to be maintained at a level somewhat lower than that of the body for spermatogenesis to occur has already been noted. High environmental temperatures may inhibit spermatogenesis and affect fertility. Rams kept in a temperate environment in summer show greater motility and fewer abnormal forms of sperm than animals exposed to high temperatures. It has also been reported that Merino sheep, which breed throughout the year, are adversely affected by the heat of the Australian summer. Matings at that time of year are followed by a lower incidence of pregnancy than at other seasons: more embryos undergo intrauterine absorption and there is a greater proportion of dwarf lambs among those developing to full term. The cooler weather of the British autumn together with its diminishing daily light may both act as favourable factors for reproductive activity at this season.

Olfaction

Experiments have clearly shown that animals influence one another's reproductive activity. For example, if pairs of male-female mice are caged together, copulation and fertilisation can be expected to follow the first oestrus of the female. Pregnancy is generally established in females left with the original stud male, or placed with other females, but Hilda Bruce found that if housed with or near strange males within 24 hours of mating pregnancy failed to occur in about 30%. Actual physical contact with the strange males was not necessary for this effect, which was observed even if the female was merely suspended in a basket from the roof of the cage containing the alien. Blocking of pregnancy did not occur if the olfactory bulbs of the female had been removed, which suggests that the inhibitory effect is most likely due to an olfactory stimulus.

Olfaction is an important sense in most mammals and female mice deprived of their sense of smell lose their regular oestrous cycles. Large numbers of female mice housed together show irregular cycles, while the introduction of a male into the group, even if isolated from the females by being confined in a basket, is followed by oestrus in most of the females within a few days. Olfactory stimuli modify reproductive cycles in other species of mammals, for example voles and sows.

Such effects mediated through olfactory receptors suggest that pheromones (ectohormones) (see p. 9) act in mammals as well as in invertebrates. Substances of this kind may seem somewhat removed from human reproductive activity, but olfactory stimuli have been shown to play a role in primates.

Noise

Auditory stimuli may exert some influence on reproductive cycles, although the strength and duration of the stimuli used experimentally has been well outside the normal range to which the animals were likely to be exposed. The sounding of a bell for one minute at ten minute intervals, day and night for two months, was associated with a considerable increase in the weight of both uterus and ovaries in rats and rabbits. Exposure of paired rats to excessive and recurrent noise was associated with a great reduction in the incidence of pregnancy, from an average of 80% in control pairs to 20%. Perhaps surprisingly the noise did not seem to interfere with copulation and ejaculation. The number of young born was decreased when females were exposed only after the mating peroid, but not if the noise was delayed until pregnancy was well established.

The increased weight of uterus and ovaries in animals exposed to what must be a stressful stimulus suggests that there had been an increase in the output of gonadotropic hormones from the pituitary gland. The adrenal cortex would also doubtless respond to stress with an increased secretion of corticoids, and indeed increase in size and activity of the adrenals was noted. Other studies however have reported a diminution of gonadotropic hormones as a response to stress, which cannot be easily reconciled with the above findings.

Nutrition

The availability of food, a prerequisite for reproductive activity in some birds, can also play a role in some mammalian species. "Flushing" of sheep, giving the ewes extra food in the breeding season, can precipitate oestrus. The composition of the diet is important and lack of a number of elements as well as chronic underfeeding may reduce fertility. Breeding tends to be more successful in populations inhabiting areas where food is abundant; malnutrition of course affects not only reproductive processes, but many other bodily functions.

The examples given indicate the kind of stimuli which may affect reproductive activity in various living creatures. Light, heat, cold and noise are fairly easy to appreciate and measure. Olfactory stimuli among others are less easy to assess, and there is no ready way of determining their strength. Also it may be difficult to distinguish between effects due to, say, olfaction from those resulting from crowding or competition for food.

The importance of any given environmental stimulus is difficult to determine even for animals. Experiments designed to determine the effect of a single factor such as light can be devised, but considerable care is necessary to ensure that only one variable is involved in producing any observed effect. Two groups of animals are necessary, one as control, the other subjected to the single variable. Genetically, the two groups should ideally be identical; conditions of housing, handling, diet, times of feeding and cleaning should all be standardised for the two groups, and other possible environmental stimuli, such as noise, temperature, humidity, should be identical for all.

MAN

Standardisation of this order can be achieved, albeit expensively, in studies of animals. It is much more difficult to derive reliable information for human beings. Light, for example, might influence human reproductive activity, but controlled experiments in which all other factors are standardised are impracticable for the number of individuals necessary to give a statistically valid result. We can analyse birth rates correlated with time of year, and hence with natural day length; but individuals are exposed to varying intensities of artificial light for varying times according to habit and the environment varies locally, as do diet, health, religious, social and other factors. All this makes a meaningful assessment of the problem where man is concerned extremely difficult. Nevertheless there is enough evidence to suggest that human reproductive processes may be susceptible to some degree of modulation by environmental conditions.

Estimates of the conception rates in human populations are based on figures for births, which are extensive and reliable for many countries. Interpretation of the significance of these figures is another matter, and it is hardly surprising that views differ. On the one hand seasonal variations of birth rates in Finland have been taken to indicate that the rate of conception in women was increased following a sunny spring, while after a dark spring the conception rate was higher later in the year. The greatest number of conceptions was said to follow about a month after the peak luminosity. A further conclusion was that the incidence of twin births reached a peak in March, nine months after the long northern days of midsummer.

On the other hand MacFarlane has argued against any appreciable photoperiodic control of human conception. A summary of demographic studies of births in many different parts of the world with greatly varying climatic conditions and seasonal fluctuations led him to suggest that temperature, not light, is the major environmental factor for women. Birth records indicate that while variations of frequency of conception are widespread, there is no close overall correlation with day length. Maximum frequency of conception in Sweden for example occurs in the long summer days, but in mid-West U.S.A. in the short winter days. Seasonal variations in the rate in Britain, where the difference between midsummer and midwinter day length exceeds six hours, are less than those in southern India, where the variation is only an hour or so. MacFarlane concludes that "thermal comfort", which is equated with spring in latitudes between 30° and 40° N in Mediterranean countries, and with early summer (45° N and above) in more northern European countries is the determining factor. Conception rates in countries with hot summers and cool winters show winter maxima, and altitude compensates for unfavourable latitudes. Making allowances for widespread air conditioning, hot seasons are associated with lower fertility.

The probable importance of temperature does not exclude the possibility that other environmental factors have some effect on human reproduction. Barometric pressure, humidity, noise, diet and the level of nutrition, as well as other factors, may all play a part.

Altitude

The environment at high altitudes is likely to differ from that of the lowlands in a number of ways notably temperature, humidity, intensity of light and ultraviolet illumination. At those extreme altitudes which are still tolerable to man, the barometric pressure and the low partial pressure of oxygen are probably the most relevant factors.

The effect on various physiological functions of living at high altitudes has been considered with particular reference to the inhabitants of the Peruvian Andes, where man and animals have lived for centuries at altitudes between 10,000 and 16,000 feet. Monge (1942) cites a certain Father Calancha who in 1639 described how the race of Spanish conquerors living in Potosi, lying at 14,000 feet, produced no offspring until many years after the city was founded. By contrast, the natives were fully fertile. He also wrote that the capital was transferred from Jauja (13,000 feet) to Lima at sea-level because domestic birds and animals did not breed at high altitude. Monge describes the various physiological changes associated with the state of chronic mountain sickness, of which infertility is only one manifestation. Adaptation may occur in due course, in effect a "cure" of the sickness and with it a return of fertility in both man and animals. Rams which had become acclimatised over a long period were fully fertile at the high altitudes, but only 50% of those brought from sea level were able to produce offspring in their first year, a figure increasing to 70% after two or three years.

Effects due to reduced atmospheric pressure may be of some relevance to aeroplane pilots. High flying aircraft are of course pressurised, but not to ground level pressures; frequent intermittent exposure to cabin altitudes lower than "normal" might induce testicular damage and adrenal changes associated with stress, with consequent effects on reproductive functions. Effects on airline stewardesses are even more likely, with the frequent changes of light-dark patterns and climate disturbing their "biological clocks" and precipitating menstrual irregularities.

How environmental factors act

Modification of reproductive cycles is predominantly brought about by a change in the pattern of secretion of the pituitary gonadotropins, which in turn modifies gonadal secretions. In view of what is known about hypothalamic control of the pituitary it is now clear that the central nervous system is involved, acting largely via the hypothalamus as a "final common path". Although the location of some of the "higher centres" which act on the hypothalamus is known, the full mechanism is not clear.

Attention has already been drawn to the importance of light as a stimulus, and many attempts have been made to demonstrate a retino-hypothalamic nervous pathway over which the effects of light might be mediated. There is recent evidence that in animals neurons of the suprachiasmatic nuclei in the anterior hypothalamus receive such an input and are concerned in the mediation of the effects of light on endocrine activity.

The pineal body (see below) is also involved in responses to light, but it is not necessarily the only extra-hypothalamic structure concerned. Specialised receptors such as the olfactory mucosa and bulbs clearly play a part in the input of other appropriate stimuli to the central nervous system, and something is known about the central pathways for these and other stimuli. Factors such as environmental temperature also presumably exert an influence via the hypothalamus.

In addition to effects mediated via the hypothalamo-pituitary-gonadal axis, the gonads may be directly influenced. The testes, as has been seen, are susceptible to local variations in temperature and also to dietary factors; deficiencies of certain vitamins and minerals can affect spermatogenesis, and some subtances have cytotoxic effects (cadmium for example can produce tubular damage). Low oxygen tension may directly damage the germinal epithelium and decrease fertility. Low levels of X-radiation can damage the germ cells in both ovaries and testes and cause genetic defects in fetuses, while high levels will destroy the germ cells and result in sterility.

THE PINEAL BODY

Even as recently as the mid-1950s, the pineal body (or gland) could not with any certainty be considered to have a role of particular importance in relation to reproductive activity. A major review, published by Kitay and Altschule in 1954, ended with the comment that "although the available physiological and clinical data justify the presumption that the gland is functional, its functions cannot yet be defined". The authors had come to this conclusion despite the fact that their bibliography listed over 1700 publications dealing specifically with the pineal.

Our knowledge today is somewhat more advanced and studies over the last fifteen years or so strongly suggest that the pineal is, if not a true endocrine gland, then at any rate closely linked to the endocrine system and that it has a particular relationship to reproductive activity. It is now regarded as a neuroendocrine transducer rather than a gland, receiving a direct nervous input and modulating, by means of one or more specific "transmitter" type substances, the activity of the pituitary-gonadal axis. Its mode of action, although not its function, can probably be compared with the adrenal medulla, which responds to direct nervous stimulation by the release of the physiologically active substances adrenaline and noradrenaline.

Anatomy

The anatomical relations of the mammalian pineal have been to some extent responsible for the long-lasting uncertainty as to whether or not it had any important function. The organ is part of the epithalamus and develops as an evagination of the roof of the diencephalon between the habenular commissure in front and the posterior commissure behind. In some species, such as the rat, the pineal body lies superficially between the posterior poles of the cerebral hemispheres and the cerebellum, above the midbrain, connected with the diencephalic roof by a long neurovascular stalk. In man the anatomical relations are comparable except that the stalk is short and the body lies between the posterior part (the splenium) of the corpus callosum above and the superior colliculi of the roof of the midbrain below (Fig. 3), and is relatively inaccessible surgically. This also applies to some of the species (i.e. dog) in which experimental pinealectomy was first attempted and as a result the central nervous system was often severely damaged, rendering difficult any assessment of the effects of removal of the pineal. Because of its anatomical relations in man any appreciable enlargement will exert direct pressure on the diencephalic-midbrain areas.

A further hindrance to pineal studies was that the structure of the body cannot be easily demonstrated by routine histological methods. It is made up of parenchymal cells (pinealocytes) and glial elements and contains nerve fibres thought to come from various sources, notably the habenular and posterior commissures. Its blood supply is not particularly rich, although the body is related to large intracranial vessels. In some species including man it appears to undergo an early degeneration characterised by gliosis, the laying down of intercellular "ground substance" and calcification.

Clinical observations

The association of the pineal with reproductive functions was initially based on observations made on patients suffering from pineal tumours. Although these are relatively uncommon by comparison with other types of intracranial tumour, some hundreds of cases have been recorded and a wide variety of histological types described. The most striking clinical finding has been an association between parenchymal tumours and sexual precocity, and about one in four reported cases of pineal tumours in children have shown such signs; reports of pineal tumours in boys far outnumber those in girls.

Speculation as to the function of the normal pineal body on the basis of clinical and pathological data is however open to error on several grounds. Firstly, as already noted its situation within the cranial cavity inevitably means that any tumour must distort and damage surrounding brain tissues as well as increase intracranial pressure, and any direct involvement of the hypothalamus by pineal lesions is inevitably associated with gross damage to other cerebral structures. Secondly, pineal tumours are by no means the only intracranial lesions associated with precocious puberty and both experimental and clinical evidence indicates that a variety of conditions involving the hypothalamus may modify the secretion of gonadotropins by the anterior pituitary. Nevertheless clinical and pathological observations have provided the basis of two main hypotheses which have been advanced to account for the undoubted association between some pineal tumours and precocious sexual development. One proposes that the pineal normally secretes a hormone which retards development until puberty, while the other suggests that the tumour indirectly stimulates the pituitary gland, damaging either by pressure or by direct involvement the zone of the hypothalamus controlling its activity.

If some of the cellular components of the organ secrete an antigonadotropic substance it might be expected that different tumours would exert different kinds of effect according to which of the component cells had given rise to the tumour. Hyperplasia of the parenchymal (secretory) elements should produce the effects of hypersecretion; but tumours of non-secreting cells, such as a glioma derived from the supporting elements, might be associated with hypofunction due to destruction of secretory cells. Only the latter type of tumour would be expected to give rise to precocious puberty; hyperplasia of the parenchymal cells would be expected to be associated with suppression of sexual development. Reports of clinical cases suggest that there is a significant association between the non-parenchymal type of tumour and sexual precocity; although hypogonadism has been noted in patients with pineal tumours, it is so infrequent as to provide no firm statistical evidence. On balance however published reports are not incompatible with the general hypothesis that the human pineal is essentially a gonadotropin-suppressing structure.

Animal studies

Although many of the earlier published reports of studies of the pineal were inconclusive, the evidence by the late 1950s was strong enough to indicate a link with gonadal function. Most experimental work was based on one of two procedures, the removal of the pineal (pinealectomy) and the administration of extracts.

Pinealectomy of young rats results in accelerated development of the ovaries or testes, while injections of pineal extracts to prepubertal guinea pigs delays the onset of puberty as judged by the time of vaginal opening. Extracts prevented compensatory hypertrophy of the remaining ovary in rats after unilateral ovariectomy, although the number of animals used was too small for an unequivocal assessment. These and similar findings provided grounds for accepting the possibility that the pineal does play some role in the endocrine regulation of the reproductive system, at any rate in young animals.

More recent studies based on several types of approach have advanced understanding of the basic ways in which the pineal may act. Electron microscopy has demonstrated its structure; histochemical and biochemical techniques have shown the presence of certain substances, and enzymes capable of their synthesis, in pineal tissue; and activity of these substances in varying the output of pituitary hormones has been proven. A further important step has been the demonstration of pathways by which the pineal may be influenced by the nervous system.

Structure

In general the pineal of submammalian species is largely made up of cells which are directly sensitive to light, and tracts of nerve fibres carry impulses resulting from photic stimulation from the organ into the diencephalic-tegmental (i.e. the thalamus-midbrain) part of the central nervous system. In the mammalian pineal the pinealocytes, which are derived phylogenetically from the photoreceptor elements of non-mammalian forms, have lost their direct sensitivity to light. Electron microscopy shows that the cell bodies extend into processes and contain organelles common to many types of cell, but they bear no particular resemblance to secretory cells of endocrine tissues. Astrocytes are also present in the pineal and in some species, including man and other primates, nerve cells occur. Blood vessels permeate the gland and nerve fibres run in the perivascular connective tissue to end either in the pericapillary spaces or directly on the processes of pinealocytes.

The nerves which innervate the body are post-ganglionic fibres of the superior cervical sympathetic ganglia and most if not all of these reach the pineal as the "nervi conarii" which pass via the tentorium cerebelli, a fibrous sheet of dura mater to which the tip of the pineal is attached. The presence of intrapineal autonomic neurons suggests the possibility of a parasympathetic innervation as well. In some species nerve fibres enter the gland via the pineal stalk, but these are probably aberrant fibres of the habenular and posterior commissures which simply pass through without termination. In mammals there is no efferent, pinealo-fugal tract of nerve fibres. Thus, in its evolution the cells of the pineal have lost their direct sensitivity to light and become transformed into secretory cells (see below) and the gland has lost those nerve fibres which in other species carry impulses from the pineal into the central nervous system, although it has a well-developed afferent (pinealo-petal) sympathetic innervation.

The effect of light on the timing of reproductive cycles in female ferrets which, exposed to additional illumination during the winter months, come into their spring oestrus early, was described on page 128. This effect of light is abolished if the pineal gland is removed before exposure begins; but oestrus is not prevented by pinealectomy and occurs in such animals at the time of the normal spring oestrus. Removal of both superior cervical ganglia has the same effect as removal of the pineal, which diminishes in size after such an operation.

Thus, although the pineal gland is no longer in mammals subject to direct photic stimulation of its sensory cells, it appears to be influenced by light. This probably acts via the retina, an accessory optic tract travelling in the median forebrain bundle in the lateral hypothalamus, the tegmentum of the midbrain, the brain stem and the upper thoracic spinal cord. Processes of preganglionic sympathetic neurons pass from the cord to the superior cervical ganglia and postganglionic fibres form the final nervous pathway to the pineal.

Mode of action

The pineal body may exert an effect on reproductive activity by means of melatonin. Melatonin is a derivative of serotonin, which is found in the pineal and in other tissues. Most of the pineal serotonin is broken down by the enzyme monoamine oxidase, but a small proportion is converted to acetyl-serotonin from which melatonin is produced by the action of the enzyme hydroxyindole-O-methyltransferase (HIOMT). It is possible to estimate the amount of this enzyme present in pineal tissue and, since it appears to be concerned specifically in the synthesis of melatonin, it serves as an indicator of pineal activity in this respect.

The reason for the attention paid to HIOMT and to melatonin springs from a number of observations of the effect of melatonin on reproductive functions in animals. For example melatonin given to young female rats delays puberty (i.e. the time of vaginal opening) and implants into the median eminence and midbrain block the rise in pituitary LH which normally follows castration. A single dose of melatonin given to rats counteracts the increased frequency of oestrus which normally follows exposure to additional light. Continuous dosage has a similar effect, while the increased frequency of oestrus reappears when the drug is withdrawn. Melatonin also raises the serotonin level of the midbrain-hypothalamus. Serotonin, or melatonin metabolites, do not have the same effects.

These observations seem in accordance with the known anti-gonadal effects of pineal extracts. Additional support comes from observations that environmental factors and experimental procedures known to influence gonadal function result in alterations in the pineal content of HIOMT and of melatonin. The pineal's content of HIOMT (it is the only site of occurrence of this enzyme) falls when animals are exposed to greater amounts of light, and rises if they are kept in the dark. Hence the synthesis of melatonin is depressed by exposure to light, and stimulated by darkness.

In summary there seem to be reasons to believe that the pineal can act as a kind of antigonadal organ, and that it may be at any rate one of the structures involved in the mediation of the effects of environment on reproductive activity. Melatonin may be the major chemical substance involved, but how it could exert its effect is still in doubt. It might act on the central nervous system and, via the hypothalamus-pituitary, modify the secretion of gonadotropin by the adenohypophysis; it could perhaps act directly on the pituitary, on peripheral nerves or directly on the gonads. Although the evidence that light may modulate human reproductive cycles is far from conclusive, there remains a possibility that the pineal may exert some role in human reproductive processes.

11

Hormones and Behaviour

Behavioural aspects of reproduction are by no means limited to mating and the subsequent incubation or gestation periods. Many species, particularly among non-mammalian vertebrates, migrate preparatory to breeding. Rowan in 1925 first showed that light-induced stimulation of the gonads of birds was associated with the migratory urge. Many species of fish migrate, some (e.g. salmon) from salt to fresh water to spawn. Among amphibia the spring migration of frogs to the spawning ponds is well know. Aggression, courtship and display commonly precede mating in many species, even in man. Nest building is a necessary prelude to egg laying in birds and some fish.

In most vertebrates development of the full range of mating display depends on the presence of gonadal hormones; male display acts as a stimulus to the secretion of gonadotropins in the females in many species and is a necessary part of the mating pattern. Incubation behaviour in birds is associated with increasing amounts of prolactin in the plasma, but there have been differences of opinion as to whether prolactin induces the behaviour, or whether the presence of eggs (a known stimulus to incubation) brings about an increasing output of prolactin by the pituitary.

In most mammals the period of sexual receptivity is limited to the oestrous phase of the reproductive cycle, at which time mating is most likely to result in fertilisation and pregnancy. This phase is usually well defined by characteristic female behaviour. There is commonly some form of presentation to the male, with lordosis and often male-like mounting activity. In rats running activity greatly increases. Such behaviour occurs in response to the action of ovarian steroids, notably oestrogens and to a lesser extent progesterone, on the central nervous system, and it is abolished by ovariectomy. Maternal behaviour during pregnancy and after parturition is also largely hormone-dependent.

Female non-human primates are willing to accept the male during a greater proportion of the cycle than other mammals. Studies in female monkeys have shown that sexual receptivity (i.e. willingness to allow a male to mate) is influenced largely by androgens rather than by "female" sex hormones. The latter however increase the sexual "attractiveness" of females to males, and act to some extent at any rate by olfactory stimuli.

Attempts have been made to determine whether or not the occurrence and extent of sexual behaviour in women can be correlated with different phases of the menstrual cycle and hence with different patterns of stimulating hormones. Published reports are often conflicting and, in any event, basic patterns of reproductive behaviour in humans have been overlaid to varying extents by social influences. In women it has been found that removal of the ovaries has little or no effect on libido; but if the adrenal glands are also removed, then libido is rapidly depressed. Apparently androgens play a major part in regulating the sexual drive via the central nervous system.

In males the influence of androgens on sexual activity is less marked. Male animals castrated before puberty will not generally mate (and also fail to develop the full range of male secondary sexual characteristics). Castration after puberty does not necessarily lead to cessation of mating behaviour, although this generally declines. Since the testicular hormones disappear within a few days of castration, persistent sexual behaviour may depend on some changes in the nervous system already induced by male hormones, and there is ample evidence that during the post-natal developmental period the establishment of characteristic patterns of sexual behaviour is hormone-dependent.

Differences in the levels of sexual activity in different individuals of any given species are marked, but the extent to which these levels are due to hormones seems to vary from one species to another. Studies of rats with high, medium and low levels of activity, castrated and treated with androgens, indicated that the amount of androgen given did not alter the previous level of activity. Guinea pigs similarly treated, however, showed levels of activity which depended on the amount of hormone given.

Sex hormone levels in male monkeys can be affected by external circumstances. Sexual stimuli have been shown to increase the serum levels of testosterone and domination by other males to lower them. It has been claimed that the level of serum androgens is reduced in men exposed to fearful or stressful situations, and disturbances of menstrual cycles in women following physical or mental stress are well documented.

Mating behaviour

We have seen (p. 128) that antiandrogens have been used to decrease libido, but on present evidence we cannot be categorical about a positive association between plasma testosterone levels and human male sexual behaviour. Experiments to assess such a correlation have yielded conflicting results. Two independent studies, each over a period of two months, have suggested a rise in plasma testosterone in association with coitus and a 10-20 day peak level of the hormone respectively. Problems of obtaining relevant blood samples, the paucity of subjects studied and the variable level of this particular hormone even from hour to hour in the blood have made interpretation even more difficult. At best one can say that there is a circadian rhythm, plasma levels being significantly higher at 8 a.m. than at 10 p.m. There is a gradual fall in circulating levels towards midnight and during early sleep, and then plasma values of testosterone rise in a series of peaks through the night to a maximum at about 8 a.m. Interestingly, the night peaks coincide with rapid eye movement (REM) sleep which is associated with vivid dreams (often of an erotic nature) and also with the known nightly cycle of penile erection. Furthermore, should a subject be awakened immediately after a period of REM sleep, he will frequently relate spectacular details which are otherwise lost to recall by the next morning.

Several workers have found no correlation between blood androgen levels and intercourse and to date there is no report of a concomitant rise in gonadotropin levels. A reasonable suggestion has been that the reported rises in plasma testosterone have been due to increased blood flow during sexual excitement and orgasm. The situation is ripe for further investigation using multiple sampling for testosterone, dihydrotestosterone, gonadotropins and their releasing hormones.

It is possible that the hormonal status of the female may have an effect on the sexuality of the male partner, and vice versa. One report records that there is a loss of ejaculation in male rhesus monkeys after administration of progesterone to their female partners. Similarly, anosmic males lost interest in their partners, but here it has been suggested that a pheromone — suitably named copulin — is implicated. There is no evidence for a human pheromone and no reports of loss of libido in the male partners of women receiving progesterone as a contraceptive, but one wonders whether the question has been seriously asked. In the few experiments that have combined data on the hormonal status of human male and female partners studied together there is a suggestion of androgen and oestrogen peaks at early and mid-cycle and a further androgen peak towards the end of the cycle, all associated with increased coital activity. During the menstrual flow, when oestrogen levels are very low in the female, there is a tendency for plasma testosterone levels to be low and for sexual desire to wane. In many societies the mores dictate less sexual activity during the menstrual flow, so that there is a built-in reticence regardless of endocrinological considerations. The peak of activity around day 5-6 of the cycle may simply be the reaction to previous enforced continence.

Efforts to associate a peak of sexual activity with mid-cycle, when conception is most likely, have not given a clear answer to this proposition. What seemed a fairly clear cut association, both in man and in sub-human primates, has now been challenged. Suggestions that ovulation in the human might be induced by coitus have led to lively argument. Investigations have shown that many anatomical and physiological changes occur in both sexes during the sexual act. These include increase in heart rate and blood pressure, changes in respiratory rate and pattern with hyperventilation, body sweating and generalised muscular tension, but particularly contraction of smooth muscle in the female perineum and the uterus, and of the smooth muscle of the epididymis, seminal vesicles, prostate and vasa in the male. The common factor would appear to be the action of the sympathetic nervous system since this could account for all these phenomena. As an individual example, contraction of the uterus during orgasm could be attributed to the action of noradrenaline on the alpha receptors of the myometrium. There is smooth muscle in the stroma of the ovary which might also contract during orgasm, facilitating ovulation. There is known to be a high conception rate in association with rape, and one would expect there to be a release of catecholamines in this distressing and stressful situation. We know that the uterus contracts during female orgasm but we can, at present, only speculate on the reaction further up the female genital tract (i.e. uterine tubes and ovaries). Possible effects of prostaglandins occurring in human semen and also in the uterus (among other sites) have already been discussed.

It is becoming clear that the female is not a naturally passive being during sexual intercourse and that events are occurring within the female genital tract which may assist the passage of spermatozoa. Vaginal lubrication and enlargement to accommodate the penis is a universal accompaniment of sexual arousal in the female. The release of catacholamines, the action of prostaglandins and oxytocin and the additional impetus of orgasm may all play a part in facilitating fertilisation. This is important if we remember that although receptivity is not restricted in the human female, the evidence suggests that ovulation occurs at mid-cycle and that both ovum and ejaculated spermatozoa have a limited viability of about 24 hours.

References and Suggested Further Reading

Austin, C. R. (1975). Sperm fertility, viability and persistence in the female tract. *J. Reprod. Fertil.,* Suppl. **22,** 75-89.

Bedford, C. A., Challis, J. R. G., Harrison, F. A. and Heap, R. B. (1972). The role of oestrogens in the onset of parturition in various species. *J. Reprod. Fertil.,* Suppl. **16,** 1-23.

Behrman, H. R. (1974). Prostaglandins in reproduction. *Archs intern. Med.* **133,** 77-84.

Besser, G. M. and Mortimer, C. H. (1974). Hypothalamic regulatory hormones: A review. *J. Clin. Path.* **27,** 173-184.

Craig. G. M. (1975). Prostaglandins in reproductive physiology. *Postgrad. med. J.* **51,** 74-84.

Davies, J. and Ryan, K. J. (1972). Comparative endocrinology of gestation. *Vitams Horm.* **30,** 223-279.

Diczfalusy, E. (1974). Endocrine functions of the human fetus and placenta. *Am. J. Obstet. Gynec.* **119,** 419-433.

Diczfalusy, E. (1974). Fetoplacental hormones and human gestation. *Basic Life Sciences.* **4,** 385-402.

Diczfalusy, E. (1968). Mode of action of contraceptive drugs. *Am. J. Obstet. Gynec.* **100,** 136-163.

Dobrowolski, W. and Hafez, E. S. E. (1971). The uterus and the control of ovarian function. *Acta. obstet. gynec. scand.,* Suppl. **12,** 5-26.

Eliasson, R. (1973). Prostaglandins and reproduction: a general survey. *J. Reprod. Fert.* **18,** 127-132.

Elstein, M. (1975). Hormonal contraception: the current situation. *The Practitioner.* **215,** 508-519.

Euler, U. S. van. (1936). On the specific vaso-dilating and plain muscle stimulating substances from accessory genital glands in man and certain animals (Prostaglandin and Vesiglandin). *J. Physiol., Lond.* **88,** 213-234.

Everitt, B. G. and Herbert, J. (1971). The effects of dexamethasone and androgens on sexual receptivity of female Rhesus monkey. *J. Endocr.* **51,** 575-588.

Ferdman, J. (1973). Survey of recent literature on the menstrual cycle and behaviour. *J. Asthma Res.* **11,** 27-35.

Fleischer, N. and Guillemin, R. (1972). Clinical applications of hypothalamic releasing factors. *Adv. internal Med.* **18,** 303-323.

Folley, S. J. (1940). Lactation. *Biol. Revs.* **15,** 421-458.

Friesen, H. G., Fourmic, P. and Desjardins, P. (1973). Pituitary prolactin in pregnancy and normal and abnormal lactation. *Clin. Obstet. Gynec.* **16,** 25-45.

Greep, R. O. (1973). Nature, role and control of the gonadotrophins. *J. Reprod. Fert.,* Suppl. **18,** 1-13.

Hall, R. and Gomez-Pan, A. (1976). The hypothalamic regulatory hormones and their clinical application. *Adv. clin. Chem.* **18,** 173-212.

Johnson, A. D., Gomes, W. R. and VanDemark, N. L. (Eds) (1970). "The Testis" Academic Press, New York, London.

Jones, G. S., Ruchsen, M. de M., Johanson, A. J., Raiti, S. and Blizzard, R. M. (1969). Elucidation of normal ovarian physiology by exogenous gonadotropic stimulation following steroid pituitary suppression. *Fert. Steril.* **20,** 14-34.

Josimovich, J. B. (1973). Placental protein hormones in pregnancy. *Clin. Obstet. Gynec.* **16,** 46-65.

Jost, A. and Picon, L. (1970). Hormonal control of fetal development and metabolism. *Adv. Metab. Disord.* **4,** 123-184.

Keye, W. R., Yuen, B. H. and Jaffe, R. B. (1973). New concepts in the physiology of the menstrual cycle. *Clinics in Endocrinology and Metabolism.* **2,** 451-467.

Kitay, J. I. and Altschule, M. D. (1954). "The Pineal Gland: A Review of the Physiologic Literature" University Press, Harvard.

Klopper, A. (1973). Endocrinological effects of oral contraceptives. *Clinics in Endocrinology and Metabolism* **2,** 489-502.

Kulin, H. E. and Reiter, E. O. (1973). Gonadotropins during childhood and adolescence: A review. *Pediatrics, Springfield* **51,** 260-271.

Liggins, G. C. (1973). Fetal influences on myometrial contractility. *Clin. Obstet. Gynec.* **16,** 148-165.

Marshall, F. H. A. (1922). "The Physiology of Reproduction" (2nd edition) Longmans Green, London.

Marshall, W. A. and Tanner, J. M. (1969). Variations in pattern of pubertal changes in girls. *Archs Dis. Childh.* **44,** 291-303.

Marshall, W. A. and Tanner, J. M. (1970). Variations in the pattern of pubertal changes in boys. *Archs Dis. Childh.* **45,** 13-23.

MacFarlane, W. V. (1974). Seasonal cycles of human conception. *Prog. Biometeorol.* **1,** 557-57.

Monge, C. (1942). Life in the Andes and chronic mountain sickness. *Science, N.Y.* **95,** 79-84.

Nalbandov, A. V. (1976). "Reproductive Physiology of Mammals and Birds"(3rd. edition.) W. H. Freeman, San Francisco.

Niswender, G. D., Menon, K. M. J. and Jaffe, R. B. (1972). Regulation of the corpus luteum during the menstrual cycle and early pregnancy. *Fert. Steril.* **23,** 432-442.

Parkes, A. S. (1963). External factors in mammalian reproduction. *Sci. Basis Med. Ann. Revs.* Athlone Press, University of London.

Pincus, G. (1955). Proc. Vth. int. conf. Planned Parenthood, Tokyo.

Reiter, E. O. and Kulin, H. E. L. (1972). Sexual maturation in the female. Normal development and precocious puberty. *Pediat. Clins. N. Am.* **19.** 3, 581-603.

Root, A. W. (1973). Endocrinology of puberty. I. Normal sexual maturation. *J. Pediat.* **83,** 1-19.

Schally, A. V., Kastin, A. J. and Arimura, A. (1972). The hypothalamus and reproduction. *Am. J. Obstet. Gynec.* **114,** 421-442.

Speroff, L. and VandeWiele, R. L. (1971). Regulation of the human menstrual cycle. *Amer. J. Obstet. Gynec.* **109,** 234-247.

Tanner, J. M. (1978). "Foetus into Man: Physical Growth from Conception to Maturity" Open Books, London.

Wurtman, R. J., Axelrod, J. and Kelly, D. E. (1968). "The Pineal". Academic Press, New York, London.

Wurtman, R. J. (1969). The pineal gland in relation to reproduction. *Am. J. Obstet. Gynec.* **104,** 320-326.

INDEX